Textbook of

Medical Bioethics, Attitude and Communication

for Medical Students

Textbook of

Medical Bioethics, Attitude and Communication

for Medical Students

Motilal C Tayade
MBBS, MD, PhD Scholar

Assistant Professor
Department of Physiology
Pravara Institute of Medical Sciences, Loni
Tal Rahata, Ahmednagar, Maharashtra

CBS Publishers & Distributors Pvt Ltd

New Delhi • Bengaluru • Chennai • Kochi • Kolkata • Mumbai
Bhopal • Bhubaneswar • Hyderabad • Jharkhand • Nagpur
• Patna • Pune • Uttarakhand • Dhaka (Bangladesh)

Textbook of
Medical Bioethics, Attitude and Communication
for Medical Students

ISBN: 978-81-239-2972-9

Copyright © Author and Publisher

First Edition: 2016

Reprint: 2020

Published by Satish Kumar Jain and produced by Varun Jain for

CBS Publishers & Distributors Pvt Ltd

4819/XI Prahlad Street, 24 Ansari Road, Daryaganj, New Delhi 110 002, India.

Ph: 23289259, 23266861, 23266867   Website: www.cbspd.com

Fax: 011-23243014   e-mail: delhi@cbspd.com; cbspubs@airtelmail.in

Corporate Office: 204 FIE, Industrial Area, Patparganj, Delhi 110 092

Ph: 4934 4934   e-mail: publishing@cbspd.com; publicity@cbspd.com

Fax: 4934 4935

Branches

- **Bengaluru:** Seema House, 2975, 17th Cross, K.R. Road, Banasankari 2nd Stage, Bengaluru 560 070, Karnataka

  Ph: +91-80-26771678/79   Fax: +91-80-26771680   e-mail: bangalore@cbspd.com

- **Chennai:** 7, Subbaraya Street, Shenoy Nagar, Chennai 600 030, Tamil Nadu

  Ph: +91-44-26680620, 26681266   Fax: +91-44-42032115   e-mail: chennai@cbspd.com

- **Kochi:** 42/1325, 1326, Power House Road, Opposite KSEB Power House, Ernakulam 682 018, Kochi, Kerala

  Ph: +91-484-4059061-65   Fax: +91-484-4059065   e-mail: kochi@cbspd.com

- **Kolkata:** 6/B, Ground Floor, Rameswar Shaw Road, Kolkata-700 014, West Bengal

  Ph: +91-33-22891126, 22891127, 22891128   e-mail: kolkata@cbspd.com

- **Mumbai:** 83-C, Dr E Moses Road, Worli, Mumbai-400018, Maharashtra

  Ph: +91-22-24902340/41   Fax: +91-22-24902342   e-mail: mumbai@cbspd.com

Representatives

• Bhopal	0-8319310552	• Bhubaneswar	0-9911037372	• Hyderabad	0-9885175004
• Jharkhand	0-9811541605	• Nagpur	0-9421945513	• Patna	0-9334159340
• Pune	0-9623451994	• Uttarakhand	0-9716462459	• Dhaka (Bangladesh)	01912-003485

Printed at Mudrak, Noida, UP, India

Contributors

Dr A U Siddhiqui
Assistant Professor, Department of Anatomy
All India Institute of Medical Sciences, Raipur, Chhattisgarh

Dr Abolee Paithankar
Intern, Pravara Institute of Medical Sciences
Loni, Maharashtra

Dr Kirankumar Jadhav
Associate Professor, Department of Surgery
BJ Medical College, Pune, Maharashtra

Dr Monika Gawali
Assistant Professor, Department of Physiology
Kashibai Navale Medical College
Pune, Maharashtra

Dr Naveen Pahade
Intern, Government Medical College
Aurangabad, Maharashtra

Dr Pinaki Wani
Department of Physiology, KJ Somaiya Medical College
Mumbai, Maharashtra

Dr Prathmesh Kamble
Assistant Professor
Department of Physiology, BJ Medical College
Pune, Maharashtra

Dr R G Latti
Professor and Head, Department of Physiology, RMC, PIMS
Loni, Maharashtra

Dr Sachin Wankhede
Associate Professor, Department of Microbiology
Kashibai Navale Medical College
Pune, Maharashtra

Dr Sanjay Lagdive
Professor, Government Dental College
Ahmedabad, Gujarat

Dr Shantanu Choudhari
Professor and Head, Department of Pedodontics
Govt Dental College, Ahmedabad, Gujarat

Dr Sunil Bhamare
Assistant Professor
Department of Microbiology, BJ Medical College
Pune, Maharashtra

Dr Sushma Lagdive
Assistant Professor, Department of Periodontia
Siddhpur Dental College and Hospital, Siddhpur
Dethali, Gujarat

Dr Vinod
Assistant Professor
Department of Physiology, MR Medical College
Gulbarga, Karnataka

Miss Pratibha Karandikar
Lecturer, Mechanical Department, PREC
Loni, Maharashtra

Preface

It gives me an immense pleasure in writing this saga of medical bioethics. Bioethics is now at the center stage of medical education. Horizontally and vertically integrated bioethics curriculum has been designed by the foundation of the UNESCO, bioethics core curriculum. This textbook is written with an intention to explain the basic concepts in medical bioethics in easier language and simple justifications. This textbook will definitely be helpful to students for easy seeding of concepts of bioethics and quick review, especially during examination period. I have tried to avoid lengthy explanation of concepts and cases associated with these facts. Definitions are designed and prepared with efforts and lots of discussions with experts and this is the highlighting aspect of this textbook. Historical aspects are edited as per requirement of students. Some facts and narrations are obtained from concerned reference books and research papers with citations. More than 800 research papers are searched and studied in writing this textbook. Most of the historical aspects included in this book are obtained from online sources, e-books, bioethics specialty journals, and other multidisciplinary biomedicals, etc. and I have provided citations and credits for them. Some topics such as guidelines declared by Medical Council of India (MCI), CPCESA Act, etc. are not edited, henceforth, not to change their meaning. I provide credits to these important organizations and their policymakers. I tried to make this textbook simple and lucid.

The undergraduate medical education program is currently modulated and designed with a goal to create medical graduate possessing requisite knowledge, skills, attitudes, values and responsiveness, so that he may function appropriately and effectively as a doctor of first contact of the community while being globally relevant. There are many new key areas recommended in the ATCOM module that are identified for implementation across the entire duration of the course. In extent of order the medical graduate is not only physician but also leader of society, communicator as well as counselor, lifelong learner and professional who is committed for the best, ethical, responsive and accountable to society. Physician is not only concerned with curative approach but also accountable for preventive care, holistic care, promotive and palliative care of community. With this background, I included chapters, viz. 'Professionalism' and 'Attitude and Communication', for competencies of the medical graduate for understanding doctor–patient relationship and responsibilities of the doctor in the community.

This textbook contains the basic principles of medical bioethics in theoretical form (foundation course) which will be helpful for MBBS students and other courses, viz. BDS, physiotherapy, nursing, and other paramedical courses. It will be also helpful for clinical practitioners for understanding basic concepts in medical bioethics.

This textbook is written on the basis of guidelines declared by UNESCO and Chair Head, Medical Bioethics, Haifa, Australia. The same guidelines are adopted by a number of universities across India.

I hope and believe this will ever be the first textbook which clearly explains the basic concepts and principles of bioethics with attitude and communication competencies required for medical students from Indian subcontinent and helpful in their academic curriculum and clinical practice.

Herewith, I express my sincere thanks and deep appreciation to Dr Balasaheb Vikhe Patil, Padmabhushan awardee, under his blessings this historical saga of writing 'Medical Bioethics' has been possible in the calm and beautiful land of Loni.

I express my sincere thanks and deep appreciation to Mr Rajendra Vikhe Patil, Chief Executive, Pravara Medical Trust, Loni, who always inspires us in every academic and research activities in our institution.

I express my sincere thanks and deep appreciation to Prof. (Dr) Russell D'Souza, Head, Asia Pacific Bioethics Programme, UNESCO Chair in Bioethics, Haifa, Australia, for his inspiration and seeding concept of medical bioethics.

I express my sincere thanks and deep appreciation to Dr Mary Mathew and Dr Princy Palatty for their inspiration and support in understanding basic concepts of medical bioethics.

I express my sincere thanks and deep appreciation to Dr Shashank Dalvi, Vice Chancellor, Pravara Institute of Medical Sciences, Loni; and Dr DS Kulkarni, Principal, Rural Medical College, Loni, for their constant inspiration.

I express my sincere thanks and deep appreciation to Dr Ramchandra G Latti, Head, Department of Physiology, and my inspiring and disciplined PhD guide, who always promote us for new horizons.

I express my sincere thanks and deep appreciation to Dr DB Phalake, Professor and Head, Department of PSM, and Coordinator, MET Unit, Rural Medical College, Loni, for his support while writing this textbook.

Herewith, I am specially very thankful to Dr Sunil Bhamare, Dr Kirankumar Jadhav, Dr Prathmesh Kamble and Dr Abolee Paithankar who are the active contributors in writing this textbook. Dr Sunil Bhamare from BJ Medical College, Pune, is my best friend initiated me to write over this topic. Dr Sunil helped me in writing two topics—animal ethics and research. Dr Kirankumar Jadhav, Associate Professor of Surgery, BJ Medical College, who helped me in writing human rights and issues concerned with euthanasia. Dr Prathmesh helped me in writing physiology section and fundamentals of medical ethics. Dr Abolee Paithankar, MBBS intern and disciplined student, helped me in writing historical aspects from human rights, euthanasia, biocentrism and immortality.

I am very thankful to my wife Pratibha who regularly inspired me. I am very thankful to my lovely son Nirav and cute baby Arohi who never troubled me during writing. Both of them act as my energy. I am very thankful to my parents who always stand behind me in every situation whenever I am disappointed.

Finally I express my sincere thanks and deep appreciation to CBS Publishers & Distributors who in a very short time accepted my script and completed necessary formalities with priority. I am also specially thankful to Mr Sitaram Shelake, Pravara Medical Book Sellers, Loni.

I always believe in hard work and blessings of God. This historical saga is written in the land of Shirdi. This work is carried out with the blessings of Sai Baba.

Finally my students are the source of my energy and inspiration and due to their constant inspiration I could write this book.

Development of curriculum is a continuous process. There is always scope for improvement, simplification of concepts, basic principles and addition of updated knowledge, so I request all my students, faculty members and those who are using this textbook, to evaluate the material and offer their valuable suggestions and criticism for improving the quality and content of this textbook.

Motilal C Tayade

Contents

25. Professionalism and MCI Regulations   133

26. The Right to Information (RTI) Act of India   143

27. Hippocratic Oath   149

28. Attitude and Communication   154

1

Medical Bioethics: Introduction

LEARNING OBJECTIVES

After reading this chapter student should:
• Be able to define bioethics, medical bioethics, autonomy, beneficence and non-maleficence
• Know areas of bioethics in practice and scope of bioethics
• Know historical aspects of bioethics
• Know well-known medical ethics cases in India and worldwide
• Understand values of medical bioethics

INTRODUCTION

Bioethics is the study of controversial ethical issues emerging from new situations due to advances in biology and medicine. Bioethics is the area concerned with ethical questions that arise in the relationships among life sciences, biotechnology and healthcare sciences, etc.

The term Bioethics (Greek bios, life; ethos, behavior) was coined in 1926 by Fritz Jahr.

In 1970, the American biochemist Van Rensselaer Potter used the term with a broader meaning including solidarity towards the biosphere, thus generating a "global ethics," a discipline representing a link between biology, ecology, medicine and human values in order to attain the survival of human beings.

The scope of bioethics can expand with advancements and inventions in healthcare sector like cloning, gene therapy, life extension therapy, human genetic engineering, astroethics, etc.

1

The National Commission for the Protection of Human Subjects of Biomedical and Behavioral Research was initially established in 1974 to identify the basic ethical principles that should underlie the conduct of biomedical and behavioral research involving human subjects.

Human experimentation thus found first area of interest of bioethics.

However, the **Belmont Report** (1979) added basic fundamental principles, viz **autonomy, beneficence and justice**.

Following Belmont Report other experts included **nonmaleficence, human dignity and the sanctity of life** to this list of cardinal values.

MEDICAL BIOETHICS

Medical bioethics is the system of moral principles that apply values and judgments to clinical practice.

Ethics is the integral part of clinical practice. Ethics deals with the choices. Ethical practices involve systemic approach in every decision making.

Medical bioethics is simply concerned with applied professional ethics, whereas bioethics appears to have worked in more expansive concerns, including the philosophy of science and issues of biotechnology.

Still, the two fields often overlap and the distinction is more a matter of style than professional consensus.

Medical bioethics shares many principles with other branches of healthcare ethics.

Religions and Fundamentals of Bioethics

Many ancient religious communities have made their own rules and guidelines on the basis of their faith, beliefs, idolism and historical events.

The Jewish, Christian, Hindu, Buddhist and Muslim faiths have developed guidelines, principles and considerable literature.

In Africa and Latin America, the debate on bioethics frequently focuses on its practical relevance in the context of underdevelopment and geopolitical power relations.

Medical Bioethics Areas in Practice

Following is the list of areas produced due to advancement in modern healthcare management system and biotechnology field.

- Abortion
- Animal rights
- Artificial insemination
- Artificial life
- Artificial womb
- Assisted suicide
- Advanced life support
- Biocentrism
- Biological patent
- Biohazards
- Biotic ethics
- Blood transfusion
- Body modification
- Brain-computer interface
- Chimeras
- Circumcision
- Cloning
- Consent
- Compulsory sterilization movement
- Contraception (birth control)
- Cryonics
- Disability
- Eugenics
- Euthanasia (human, non-human animal)
- Exorcism
- Faith healing
- Feeding tube
- Gene theft
- Gene therapy
- Genetically modified food
- Genetically modified organism

- Genetically assisted products
- Genomics
- Great Ape Project
- Hypnotherapy
- Human cloning
- Human enhancement
- Human experimentation in the United States
- Human genetic engineering
- Iatrogenesis
- Infertility treatments
- Life extension
- Life support
- Life support therapy
- Lobotomy
- Medicalization
- Medical malpractice
- Medical research
- Medical pharama research
- Medical torture
- Medical confidentiality
- Medical negligence
- Mediation therapy
- Moral obligation of doctor
- Moral status of animals
- Nanomedicine technology
- Nazi human experimentation
- Ordinary and extraordinary care
- Organ donation
- Organ transplant
- Pain management
- Parthenogenesis
- Patients' Bill of Rights
- Pharmaceutical research
- Placebo

- Pharmacogenetics
- Political abuse of psychiatry
- Population control methods
- Prescription drug prices in the United States
- Procreative beneficence
- Professional ethics
- Psychosurgery
- Quality of life (healthcare)
- Quaternary prevention
- Recreational drug use
- Reproductive rights
- Reprogenetics
- Sex reassignment therapy
- Sperm and egg donation
- Spiritual drug use
- Stem cell research
- Suicide
- Surrogacy
- Three-parent babies
- Transexuality
- Transhumanism
- Transplant trade
- Vaccination controversy
- Xenotransfusion
- Xenotransplantation
- Yoga

Historical Aspects of Medical Bioethics

The first documented code of medical ethics, Formula **Comitis Archiatrorum**, was published in the 5th century. In the early modern period, the field is indebted to Muslim medicine such as Ishaq ibn Ali al-Ruhawi (who wrote the Conduct of a Physician, the first book dedicated to medical ethics) and Muhammad ibn Zakariya ar-Razi (known as Rhazes in the West), Jewish thinkers such as Maimonides, Roman Catholic scholastic thinkers such as Thomas Aquinas, and the case-oriented analysis (casuistry) of Catholic moral theology.

These traditions continue in Catholic, Islamic and Jewish medical ethics.

By the 18th and 19th centuries, medical ethics emerged as a more self-conscious discourse.

In England, Thomas Percival, a physician, crafted the first modern code of medical ethics.

In 1815, the Apothecaries Act was passed by the Parliament of the United Kingdom. It introduced mandatory regulations and formal qualifications for the apothecaries of the day under the license of the Society of Apothecaries. This was the beginning of regulation of the medical profession in the UK.

In 1847, the American Medical Association introduced and announced its first code of ethics, with this being based in large part upon Percival's work.

Well-known medical ethics cases

- Aruna Shanbaug case (India)—Euthanasia
- Milgram experiment
- Radioactive iodine experiments
- Right of Information Act (RTI Act) of India
- The Monster study
- Plutonium injections
- The David Reimer case
- Burning migration issues
- Human rights activities in worldwide scenario
- Animal rights activists work
- The Stanford Prison Experiment
- Tuskegee syphilis experiment
- Willowbrook State School
- Movement of compulsory sterilization—international level
- Yanomami blood sample collection
- Darkness in El Dorado
- Albert Kligman's dermatology experiments
- Deep sleep therapy

- Doctors' trial
- Greenberg vs. Miami Children's Hospital Research Institute
- Henrietta Lacks
- Human radiation experiments
- Jesse Gelsinger
- Moore vs. Regents of the University of California
- Surgical removal of body parts to try to improve mental health
- Medical experimentation on Black Americans

Values in Medical Bioethics

Medical bioethics is based on the framework postulated by Tom Beauchamp and James Childress.

It is based on four fundamental principles which are to be judged against each other.

The four principles are:

1. **Respect for autonomy:** The patient has the right to refuse or choose their treatment. This is most important principle of medical bioethics. The principles of autonomy are based on the rights of individuals to self-determination. Nowadays clinical practice is shifted as more patient oriented, the value of autonomy increased. Respect for autonomy is the basis for informed consent and advance directives.

2. **Beneficence:** A practitioner should act in the best interest of the patient. Every activity or treatment plan should involve objectives concern with patient beneficence rather than doctor or any other.

3. **Non-maleficence:** "First, do no harm". This is the third important principle of medical bioethics.

4. **Justice:** Concerns the distribution of scarce health resources, and the decision of who gets what treatment.

2

Autonomy, Beneficence and Non-maleficence

LEARNING OBJECTIVES

After reading this chapter student should:
- Be able to define autonomy, beneficence and non-maleficence
- Understand basic concepts of autonomy, beneficence and non-maleficence
- Understand the basic fundamental framework of principle of bioethics formed by James Childress and Tom Beauchamp.
- Understand double effect and principle of double effect in bioethics
- Understand practical conflicts between autonomy and beneficence/non-maleficence
- Know about fundamental ethical issues and unnecessary surgical procedures in clinical practice

INTRODUCTION

The principles of autonomy are based on the right of individuals to self-determination.

Nowadays clinical practice is shifted more patient oriented, the value of autonomy increased. Respect for autonomy is the basis for informed consent and advance directives. By autonomy it is patient right what he wants. Refusal to treatment or any investigation or any surgical procedure is sole autonomy of any patient.

Autonomy is a general indicator of health.

By considering autonomy as a basic parameter for healthcare, the medical and ethical perspectives both benefit from the implied reference to health.

It is urged by psychiatrists and psychologists to evaluate patient's capacity for making life-and-death decisions at critical level. Hence right to refuse a treatment should be considering fact under all observations and good faith. This is highly challenging with mental illness patients and pediatric age patients. In that cases, psychiatrists and psychologists play an important role in protecting rights of patient in these cases respectively mentally ill patients and children. In other cases it is clinician's first priority to maintain the autonomy of patient irrespective to other values. Most of the situations patient is not in a situation to take right decision. That time it is clinician's moral responsibility to explain the situation to his patient and relatives.

Otherwise, refuse a treatment is sole autonomy of any patient.

Beneficence

The action or act that promotes well-being of others is known as beneficence.

In medical scenario this implies treatment should be allotted by clinician in the best interest of patients. Here treatment should be allotted in best patient interest rather than doctors himself. Very unfortunately patient beneficence is not regularly follows in our clinical practice. Cut practice from specialty doctors known for referral services, cut from laboratories for investigations resulting practices of unnecessary list of investigations and cut from medical store resulting in prescription of unnecessary costly medicines.

James Childress and Tom Beauchamp in *Principle of Biomedical Ethics* (1978) identifies beneficence as one of the core values of healthcare ethics. Some scholars, such as Edmund Pellegrino, argue that beneficence is the only fundamental principle of medical ethics. They argue that healing should be the sole purpose of medicine, and that endeavors like cosmetic surgery and euthanasia fall beyond its purview. Every decision what clinician finalize for his patient, along with autonomy, it should be always patient benefit oriented or reducing his pain.

NON-MALEFICENCE

The concept of non-maleficence is embodied by the phrase, **"first, do no harm,"** or the Latin, *primum non nocere*.

In clinical practice doctor's goal should be not to harm patients, than to do them good. Before application of any treatment plan, the clinician should be fully evaluated the ongoing effects and possibilities of harm in the future. "We do our best but patient died" such saying that than to do well; it is also important to know how likely it is that treatment will harm a patient.

In practice, however, many treatments carry some risk or harm. In some circumstances, e.g. in desperate situations where the outcome without treatment will be grave, risky treatments that stand a high chance of harming the patient will be justified, as the risk of not treating is also very likely to do harm. So the principle of non-maleficence is not absolute, and balances against the principle of beneficence (doing good), as the effects of the two principles together often give rise to a double effect.

Depending on the cultural consensus conditioning (expressed by its religious, political and legal social system) the legal definition of non-maleficence differs. Violation of non-maleficence is the subject of medical malpractice litigation. Regulations therefore differ over time, per nation.

Double Effect and Principle of Double Effect

Double effect refers to two types of consequences that may be produced by a single action, and in medical ethics area, it is usually regarded as the combined effect of beneficence and non-maleficence.

A commonly cited example of this phenomenon is the use of morphine or other analgesic in the dying patient. Such use of morphine can have the beneficial effect of easing the pain and suffering of the patient while simultaneously having the maleficent effect of shortening the life of the patient through suppression of the respiratory system.

Conflicts between Autonomy and Beneficence/non-maleficence

Autonomy can come into conflict with beneficence when patients disagree with decision of clinician or recommendations that healthcare professionals believe are in the patient's best interest. When the patient's interests conflict with the patient's welfare, different societies settle the conflict in a wide range of manners. In general, Western medicine defers to the wishes of a mentally competent patient to make his own decisions, even in cases where the medical team believes that he is not acting in his own best interests. However, many other societies prioritize beneficence over autonomy.

Examples include when a patient does not want a treatment because of, for example, religious or cultural views. In the case of euthanasia, the patient, or relatives of a patient, may want to end the life of the patient. Also, the patient may want an unnecessary treatment, as can be the case in hypochondria or with cosmetic surgery; here, the practitioner may be required to balance the desires of the patient for medically unnecessary potential risks against the patient's informed autonomy in the issue.

A doctor may want to prefer autonomy because refusal to please the patient's will would harm the doctor–patient relationship. Individuals' capacity for informed decision making may come into question during resolution of conflicts between autonomy and beneficence. The role of surrogate medical decision makers is an extension of the principle of autonomy.

On the other hand, autonomy and beneficence/non-maleficence may also overlap. For example, a breach of patients' autonomy may cause decreased confidence for medical services in the population and subsequently less willingness to seek help, which in turn may cause inability to perform beneficence.

The principles of autonomy and beneficence/non-maleficence may also be expanded to include effects on the relatives of patients or even the medical practitioners, the overall population and economic issues when making medical decisions.

For example, when any pregnant lady admitted in hospital in emergency and doctors plan for cesarean section as emergency cause, should be medically justified by doctors. Either interest for the sake of saving the baby or mother, the doctors' every activity or decision should be in favor of patient rather than any personal.

RESPECT FOR HUMAN RIGHTS

The Universal Declaration of Human Rights (1948) was the first major document to define human rights.

Medical doctors have an ethical duty to protect the human rights and human dignity of the patient, so the advent of a document that defines human rights has had its effect on medical ethics.

FUNDAMENTAL ETHICAL ISSUES AND UNNECESSARY SURGICAL PROCEDURES

Performing unnecessary surgical procedures is inconsistent with ethical practice because all surgical procedures bear some degree of risk. It is a major betrayal of the surgeon's paramount obligation to place the patient's best interests first in therapeutic decisions. Every year millions of patients go under knife, but many of them are enduring great pain and shelling out thousands and dollars for surgeries they don't really need. The estimated figure for the unnecessary surgical operations varies from 30 to 70%. The healthcare providers who perform surgeries simply because of profit. It is surgeon's moral responsibility to do best for patient and think whether it is appropriate for a particular patient or not. Medical justification and desire of patient and qualification of surgeon for that operative is another important ethical issue. It is not justifiable to do unnecessary surgical operations only for the sake of benefits to hospitals. According to fundamental code of ethics always consider first the well-being of the patient. The patient being treated at the time must be the physician's primary concern. Informed consent provides adequate information about the risks, benefits, and alternatives before any surgery. Performing unnecessary surgery violates rules of fundamental code of ethics. It may be a basis for malpractice liability or tort actions for fraud and battery. It may be difficult to prove which cases are unnecessary. But unnecessary surgery is that which is clearly medically unjustifiable when the risks and costs exceed the likely therapeutic benefits to the patient based on the patient's lifestyle requirements.

Most Codes of Medical Ethics now Require Respect for the Human Rights of the Patient

According to UNESCO, "Declarations are another means of defining norms, which are not subject to ratification. Like recommendations, they set forth universal principles to which the community of States wished to attribute the greatest possible authority and to afford the broadest possible support."

UNESCO adopted the Universal Declaration on Human Rights and Biomedicine to advance the application of international human rights law in medical ethics.

The Declaration provides special protection of human rights for incompetent persons.

In applying and advancing scientific knowledge, medical practice and associated technologies, human vulnerability should be taken into account. Individuals and groups of special vulnerability should be protected and the personal integrity of such individuals respected.

In conclusion, the **autonomy** is the right provided to the patient, simultaneously doctor has to obey the principles of **beneficence** and **non-maleficence** that means he has to provide best treatment to his patient and see his patient should not suffer any harm during the treatment. The base of medical ethics stands on this conclusion which extends with provision of **justice**. Patient justice is the first duty of any doctor.

Tom Beauchamp and James Childress framed their model of medical bioethics on this concept and proposed these four parameters as *basic fundamental principles of medical bioethics.*

3

Medical Confidentiality

LEARNING OBJECTIVES

After reading this chapter student should:

- Be able to define medical confidentiality
- Understand concepts of confidentiality and medical confidentiality
- Understand concept of breach of confidentiality
- Know codes and theories of ethics concerned with medical confidentiality

INTRODUCTION

Confidentiality is a binding fact that limits restrictions on specific information to disclose to third person or organization, etc.

Confidentiality in clinical practice plays a vital role. When patient discloses his private experience with doctor, his investigation reports, his any form of diagnosis, his any personal information in interest of societal cause, etc. doctors should bind not to disclosure any such record under the provision of medical confidentiality.

Medical confidentiality is an important extended principle of medical bioethics along with informed consent. Many countries along with India has made this a legal provision in their laws.

In medical bioethics, **medical confidentiality** is the most important applied principle after the four basic traditional principles suggested by Tom Beauchamp and James Childress.

DEFINITION OF MEDICAL CONFIDENTIALITY

Medical confidentiality is an issue commonly applied to information shared between doctors and patients. Legal protections prevent doctors from revealing certain discussions with patients, even under oath in court. Actually confidentiality comes as specially cornerstone of patient–doctor relationship. Respect for patient privacy, encouraging him to seek care and preventing discrimination on the basis of medical condition are the basic facts included in medical confidentiality.

The rule dates back to at least the Hippocratic Oath, which reads: Whatever, in connection with my professional service, or not in connection with it, I see or hear, in the life of men, which ought not to be spoken of abroad, I will not divulge, as reckoning that all such should be kept secret.

Traditionally, medical ethics has viewed the duty of confidentiality as a relatively non-negotiable tenet of medical practice.

Confidentiality is mandated in America by HIPAA laws, specifically the Privacy Rule, and various state laws, some more rigorous than HIPAA. However, numerous exceptions to the rules have been carved out over the years. In India there is a list of number of laws suggested by Indian Medical Council under **professional negligence** and **confidentiality of patients**. Medical Council of India has also been clearly stated regulations and provisions for misconduct and ethics. The details are discussed in Chapter 25.

Confidentiality is challenged in cases where there seen involving the diagnosis of a sexually transmitted disease in a patient who refuses to expose the diagnosis to a spouse, and in the termination of a pregnancy in an underage patient, without the knowledge of the patient's parents.

There are some important exceptions to confidentiality, namely where it conflicts with the clinician's duty to warn or duty to protect. This includes instances of suicidal behavior or homicidal plans, child abuse, elder abuse and dependent adult abuse, etc.

Nowadays medical confidentiality is one of the most important issues concerns with doctor–patient relationship.

Maintaining confidentiality of patient documents, diagnosis and other personal disclosure should be priority of any clinician. Failure of such cases has lawfully under provision of medical negligence in India.

Breach of Confidentiality

Breach of confidentiality is a concept, when one promises to keep a person's information private, but breaks that promise. Disclosure is making information about a person more accessible in a way that harms the subject of the information, regardless of how the information was collected or the intent of making it available. Exposure is a special type of disclosure in which the information disclosed is emotional to the subject or taboo to share, such as revealing their private life experiences, their nudity, or perhaps private body functions. Increased accessibility means advertising the availability of information without actually distributing it, as in the case of doxxing. Blackmail is making a threat to share information, perhaps as part of an effort to coerce someone. Appropriation is an attack on the personhood of someone, and can include using the value of someone's reputation or likeness to advance interests which are not those of the person being appropriated. Distortion is the creation of misleading information or lies about a person.

More details regarding breach of confidentiality are discussed with privacy.

Many patients are familiar with the idea of confidentiality as an integral part of the professional code of ethics in the legal, medical, and mental health fields. The information shared with doctor should be protected by him is sole requirement expected from any patients.

Medical confidentiality is recorded concept since back from Hippocratic Oath, but there are many updated versions of confidentiality, defined by various medical associations around the world. Recent years have muddied our understanding of medical confidentiality. Developments in technology have challenged our traditional understanding of "personal" information and privacy.

CODES AND THEORIES OF ETHICS

The physician's duty to keep patient information confidential dates back at least to the earliest codes of medical ethics. The Hippocratic Oath, for example, requires the physician to promise that "What I may see or hear in the course of the treatment or even outside of the treatment in regard to the life of men, which on no account one must spread abroad, I will keep to myself holding such things shameful to be spoken about."

More modern ethical codes also include statements on confidentiality. The World Medical Organization's Declaration of Geneva and the International Code of Medical Ethics both instruct the physician to maintain confidentiality, even after the patient's death. The American Medical Association's Code of Medical Ethics states that the information disclosed to the physician during the course of the relationship between the physician and patient is confidential to the greatest possible degree.

Ethical theories provide many different ways to view confidentiality laws. The doctor should rethink before exposing any information by any means or to any third party. He should always first think about his duty towards patient, patient's expectations from him, etc. However in situations that may hardens others or during some lawful help, doctor should reveals these facts or issues with honest intention and morally without any fear or wrong intention.

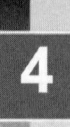

4

Nuremberg Code

LEARNING OBJECTIVES

After reading this chapter student should:

• Be able to understand history and concept of Nuremberg Code
• Know Nuremberg code–10 points
• Understand concept and issue of Declaration of Helsinki
• Know various updates and revisions involved in Declaration of Helsinki

INTRODUCTION

The **Nuremberg Code** is an official list of research ethics principles, rules and regulations for human experimentation set as a result of the Subsequent Nuremberg Trials at the end of the Second World War.

On August 20, 1947, the judges stated their verdict in the "Doctors' Trial" against Karl Brandt and 22 others.

These trials concentrated on doctors involved in the human experiments in camps. The suspects were involved in over 3,500,000 sterilizations of German citizens. The trials began on December 9, 1946 in Nuremberg, Germany and were led exclusively by the United States. Harry Truman approved these trials in January 1946. Most of the suspects escaped punishment for their crimes. Several of the accused argued that their experiments differed a little from pre-war ones and that there was no law that differentiated between legal and illegal experiments.

In May of the same year, Dr. Leo Alexander had submitted to the Counsel for War Crimes six points defining legitimate medical research. The trial verdict adopted these points and added an extra four.

The ten points constituted the "Nuremberg Code".

Although the legal force of the document was not established and it was not incorporated directly into either the American or German law, the Nuremberg Code and the related Declaration of Helsinki are the basis for the Code of Federal Regulations Title 45 Volume 46, which are the regulations issued by the United States Department of Health and Human Services governing federally funded human subjects research in the United States.

In addition, the Nuremberg code has also been incorporated into the law of individual states such as California and other countries.

NUREMBERG CODE—10 POINTS

1. For any participation as volunteer in any research activity or project or trial, is required voluntary, well-informed, understanding consent in a full legal capacity of his own.

2. The experiment should aim at positive results for society that cannot be procured in some other way.

3. It should be based on previous knowledge that justifies the experiment in documentary form.

4. The experiment should be set up in a way that avoids unnecessary physical and mental suffering and injuries.

5. It should not be conducted when there is any reason to believe that it implies a risk of death or any disabling injury.

6. The risks of the experiment should be in proportion to (that is, not exceed) the expected humanitarian benefits.

7. Preparations and facilities must be provided that adequately protect the subjects against the experiment's risks.

8. The staff that conduct or take part in the experiment must be fully trained and scientifically well and sufficient qualified.

9. The human subjects must be free to quit at any point when they feel physically or mentally unable to continue as subject in concerned research work.

10. Medical staff must stop the experiment at any point when they notice that continuation would be harmful.

THE DECLARATION OF HELSINKI

The **Declaration of Helsinki** is a list of ethical principles regarding human experimentation developed for the medical community by the World Medical Association (WMA).

It is widely regarded as the cornerstone document on human research ethics.

It is not a legally binding document under the international law, but instead draws its specific authority from the degree to which it has been codified in, or influenced, national or regional legislation and regulations.

The Declaration was originally adopted on June 1964 in Helsinki, Finland, and has since undergone seven revisions (the most recent at the General Assembly in October 2013) and two clarifications, growing considerably in length from 11 paragraphs in 1964 to 37 in the 2013 version. The Declaration is an important document in the history of research ethics as it is the first significant effort of the medical community to regulate research itself, and forms the basis of most subsequent documents.

Prior to the 1947 Nuremberg Code there was no generally accepted code of conduct governing the ethical aspects of human research, although some countries, notably Germany and Russia, had national policies. The Declaration developed the ten principles first stated in the Nuremberg Code, and tied them to the Declaration of Geneva (1948), a statement of physicians' ethical duties. The Declaration more specifically addressed to clinical research, reflecting changes in medical practice from the term 'Human Experimentation' used in the Nuremberg Code. A notable change from the Nuremberg Code was a relaxation of the conditions of consent, which was 'absolutely essential' under Nuremberg. Now doctors were asked to obtain consent 'if at all possible' and research was allowed without proper and valid consent where proxy consent, such as a legal guardian, was available.

REVISION OF DECLARATION OF HELSINKI

First Revision (1975)

The 1975 revision was almost twice the length of the original. It clearly stated that "concern for the interests of the subject must always prevail over the interests of science and society." It also introduced the concept of oversight by an 'independent committee' (Article I.2) which became a system of Institutional Review Boards (IRB) in the US, and research ethics committees or ethical review boards in other countries.

Second to Fourth Revisions (1975-2000)

Subsequent revisions between 1975 and 2000 were relatively minor, so the 1975 version was effectively governed research over a quarter of a century of relative stability.

Fifth Revision (2000)

Following the fourth revision in 1996 pressure began to build almost immediately for a more fundamental approach to revising the declaration. The later revision in 2000 would go on to require monitoring of scientific research on human subjects to assure ethical standards were being met.

Additional Principles

The most controversial revisions (Articles 29, 30) were placed in this new submitted category. These predictably were those that like the fourth revision were related to the ongoing debate in international health research. The discussions finalize that there was felt a need to send a strong signal that exploitation of poor populations as a means to an end, by research from which they would not definitely benefit, was unacceptable. In this sense the Declaration endorsed ethical universalism.

Sixth Revision (2008)

The sixth revision cycle appeared in May 2007. This consisted of a call for submissions, completed in August 2007. The terms of references included only a limited revision compared to 2000.

In November 2007 a draft revision was issued for consultation till February 2008, and led to a workshop in Helsinki in March.

Seventh Revision (2013)

The revised declaration of 2013 highlights the need to disseminate research results, including negative and inconclusive studies and also includes a requirement for treatment and compensation for injuries related to research. In addition, the updated version is felt to be more relevant to limited resource settings—specifically addressing the need to ensure access to an intervention if it is proven effective.

5

Privacy

LEARNING OBJECTIVES

After reading this chapter student should:
• Be able to define privacy, invasion and intrusion
• Understand the basic classification of privacy
• Understand the concept "Right to be left alone"
• Understand concept of personal privacy, information privacy, internet privacy and medical privacy
• Know about theories of privacy and privacy control
• Know about concept of yellow journalism
• Know about privacy laws in India
• Understand implication of privacy in clinical practice

INTRODUCTION

Privacy (from Latin: *privatus*) is defined as the ability of an individual or group to seclude themselves, or information about themselves, and thereby express themselves selectively.

Privacy may specially concerned with the form of bodily integrity in medical bioethics.

The concept of universal individual privacy is a modern construct associated with Western culture, British and North Americans in specific, and remained virtually unknown in some cultures until current times. According to some researchers, this concept sets Anglo-American culture apart even from Western European cultures such as French, Italian, etc. Most cultures, however, recognize the natural ability of an individual's to withhold certain parts of their personal information.

Therefore, in conclusion a privacy in broader sense concern with personal information.

TYPES OF PRIVACY

After searching through literature privacy can be easily classified into:
1. The right to be let alone
2. Limited access
3. Secrecy, or the option to conceal any information from others
4. Control over others' use of information about oneself
5. The idea of personhood
6. Intimacy

1. Right to be let alone

In 1890 the United States jurists Samuel D. Warren and Louis Brandeis wrote **The Right to Privacy**, an article in which they stated for the "right to be let alone", using that phrase as definition of privacy.

There is extensive debate over the meaning of being "let alone", and among other ways, it has been interpreted to mean the right of a person to choose seclusion from the attention of others if they wish to do so, and the right to be immune from scrutiny or being observed in private settings, such as one's own home, etc.

2. Limited access

Person's specific ability to participate in group or society without having other individuals and organizations collect information about them known as limited access.

Privacy may be stated as one of the systems for limiting access to one's personal information.

Edwin Lawrence Godkin wrote that "nothing is better worthy of legal protection than private life, or, in other words, the right of every man to keep his affairs to himself, and to decide for himself to what extent they shall be the subject of public observation and discussion."

3. Secrecy

Privacy may be used as term synonymous with secrecy. Richard Posner said that privacy is the right of people to "conceal information about themselves that others might use to their disadvantage".

4. Personhood

It is assumed that privacy is considered as one of fundamental aspects of personhood. It is obvious natural process of thinking in our human being that some information should be concealed. Privacy may be born due to such urge in human being and opted as one of the fundamental rights of human. In further extension it may be said that privacy may be extended as basic fundamental right due to natural will of human to maintain of individual identity. Hence we can conclude privacy be resulting from natural thought process of personhood.

5. Intimacy

There is a large number of concepts which explains relationship with other human being known as intimacy. In association with intimacy human may willfully discloses much personal information to his partner. It is very interesting thought process of human when he protects his specific information as personal; simultaneously he discloses same information to any specific person only. It is obvious observed natural tendency in human. James Rachels advanced this notion by writing that privacy matters because "there is a close connection between our ability to control who has access to us and to information about us, and our ability to create and maintain different sorts of social relationships with different people."

Personal Privacy

It is natural strong sense in any human as personal privacy mainly in relation to the exposure of their body to others. This is an aspect of personal modesty. A person will go to extreme lengths to protect this personal modesty, the main pattern being the wearing of clothes. Other ways include erection of walls, fences, screens, use of cathedral glass, partitions, by maintaining a distance, besides other ways. People who go to those lengths expect that their privacy will be respected by others. At the same time, people are ready to expose themselves in acts of physical intimacy, but these are confined to exposure in circumstances and of persons of their choosing. Even a discussion of those circumstances is regarded as intrusive and typically unwelcome.

It is very interesting thought that how to match both concepts, privacy and intimacy.

Physical privacy may be a matter of cultural sensitivity, personal dignity, and/or shyness. There may also be concerns about safety, if for example, one is wary of becoming the victim of crime or stalking. Civil inattention is a process whereby individuals are able to maintain their privacy within a crowd.

Informational Privacy

Information privacy refers to the newer relationship between technology and the legal right to, or public expectation of, privacy in the collection and sharing of data about one's self. Privacy concerns exist wherever uniquely identifiable data relating to a person or persons are collected and stored, in digital form or any other means, etc. In some cases these concerns refer to how data are collected, stored, and associated. In other cases the issue is who is given proper and suitable access to information. Other issues include whether an individual has any ownership rights to data about them, and/or the right to view, verify, and challenge that information.

Various types of personal information are often associated with privacy concerns. Information plays an important role in the decision-action process, which can lead to problems in terms of privacy and availability. First, it allows people to see all the options and suitable alternatives available. Secondly, it allows people to choose which of the best options would be best for that situation. An information landscape consists of the information, its location in the so-called network, as well as its availability, awareness, and usability. Yet the set-up of the information landscape means that information that is available in one place may not be available somewhere else. This can lead to a privacy situation that leads to questions regarding which people have the power to access and use certain information, who should have that power, and what provisions govern it. For number of reasons, individuals may object to personal information such as their religion, sexual orientation, political affiliations, or personal activities being revealed, perhaps to avoid discrimination, personal embarrassment, or damage to their professional reputations.

Internet Privacy

Internet privacy is the ability to determine what information one reveals or withholds about oneself over the internet, who has access to such information, and for what purposes one's information may or may not be used. For example, webusers may be concerned to discover that many of the websites which they visit collect, store, and possibly share personally identifiable information about them. Similarly, internet email users generally consider their emails to be private and hence would be concerned if their email was being accessed, read, stored or forwarded by third parties without their consent.

Medical Privacy

Medical privacy, i.e. protected health information [OCR/HIPAA] allows a person to withhold his medical records and other information from others, perhaps because of fears that it might affect his insurance coverage or employment, or to avoid the embarrassment caused by revealing medical conditions or treatments. Medical information could also reveal other aspects of one's personal life, such as sexual preferences or proclivity. A right to sexual privacy enables individuals to acquire and use contraceptives without family, community or legal sanctions.

HISTORICAL ASPECTS

Along with advancement in technologies, the routine way by which privacy is protected and violated has changed. In the case of some technologies, such as the printing press or the internet, the increased ability to share information can lead to new ways in which privacy can be breached. It is generally agreed that the first publication advocating privacy in the United States was the article by Samuel Warren and Louis Brandeis, "The Right to Privacy" (1890), that was written largely in response to the increase in newspapers and photographs made possible by printing technologies.

Theories of Privacy and Privacy Control

1. The **Invasion Paradigm** states privacy violation as the hostile actions of a wrongdoer who causes direct harm to an individual. This is just reactive view of privacy protection as it waits until there is a violation before acting to protect the violated individual, sometimes through criminal punishments for those who invaded the privacy of others.

2. The **Secrecy Paradigm** states a privacy invasion as someone's concealed information or hidden world being revealed through surveillance.

3. The **Negative Freedom Paradigm** views privacy as freedom from invasion rather than a right, going against the more popular view of a "right to privacy."

4. The **Inaccessibility Paradigm** states that privacy is the state where something is completely inaccessible to others.

Building from this and other historical precedents, Daniel J. Solove presented another classification of actions which are harmful to privacy, including collection of information which is already somewhat public, processing of information, sharing information, and invading personal space to get private information.

Collecting Information

In the context of harming privacy, information collection means gathering whatever information can be obtained by doing something to obtain it. Surveillance is an example of this, when someone decides to begin watching and recording someone or something, and interrogation is another example of this, when someone uses another person as a source of information.

Aggregating Information

It can happen that privacy is not harmed when information is available, but that the harm can come when that information is collected as a set, then processed in a way that the collective reporting of pieces of information encroaches on privacy.

Information Dissemination

Information dissemination is an attack on privacy when information which was shared in confidence is shared or threatened to be shared in a way that harms the subject of the information.

Breach of confidentiality is when one entity promises to keep a person's information private, and then breaks that said promise.

Disclosure is making information about a person more accessible in a way that harms the subject of the information, regardless of how the information was collected or the intent of making it available. Exposure is a special type of disclosure in which the information disclosed is emotional to the subject or taboo to share, such as revealing their private life experiences, their nudity, or perhaps private body functions. Increased accessibility means advertising the availability of information without actually distributing it, as in the case of doxxing. Blackmail is making a threat to share information, perhaps as part of an effort to coerce someone. Appropriation is an attack on the personhood of someone, and can include using the value of someone's reputation or likeness to advance interests which are not those of the person being appropriated. Distortion is the creation of misleading information or lies about a person.

Invasions

Invasion of privacy is a different issue from the collecting, aggregating, and disseminating information because those three are a misuse of available data, whereas invasion is an attack on the right of individuals to keep personal secrets. An invasion is an attack in which that information, whether intended to be public or not, is captured in a way that insults the personal dignity and right to private space of the person whose data is taken.

An **intrusion** is any unwanted entry into a person's private personal space and solitude for any reason, regardless of whether data is taken during that breach of space. "Decisional interference" is when an entity somehow injects itself into the personal decision making process of another person, perhaps to influence that person's private decisions but in any case doing so in a way that disrupts the private personal thoughts that a person has.

RIGHT TO PRIVACY

In North America, Samuel D. Warren and Louis D. Brandeis wrote that privacy is the "right to be let alone" (Warren and Brandeis, 1890) focuses on protecting individuals. This citation was a response to recent technological developments, such as photography, internet and sensationalist journalism, also known as **yellow journalism.**

Privacy rights are inherently intertwined with information technology.

In his widely cited dissenting opinion in Olmstead vs. United States (1928), Brandeis relied on thoughts he developed in his Harvard Law Review article in 1890. But in his dissent, he now changed the focus whereby he urged making personal privacy matters more relevant to constitutional law, going so far as saying "the government [was] identified . . . as a potential privacy invader." He writes, "Discovery and invention have made it possible for the Government, by means far more effective than stretching upon the rack, to obtain disclosure in court of what is whispered in the closet."

Privacy may be considered as fundamental human right and its societal value should be prominently underlined.

Amitai Etzioni suggests a communitarian approach to privacy.

To attain it as our moral culture should be in sharing form. Government as single perceptive is not sufficient in regulating privacy. Nowadays due to technological expansions and our dependence over the online information raises new issues in privacy. Sitting from any office or home and working on laptop or computer is not safe by any means. The hackers may collect every information and sell them in the market and makes money is the routine practice in the cyber world. The bank account hackers may empty your account within minutes. Your every digital information can be stolen by any expert and misuse it in the future.

The human right to privacy has precedent in the United Nations Declaration of Human Rights: "Everyone has the right to freedom of opinion and expression; this right includes freedom to hold opinions without interference and to seek, receive and impart information and ideas through any media and regardless of frontiers." Shade believes that privacy should be considered from a people-centered perspective, and not through the marketplace.

The United Nations Universal Declaration of Human Rights says "No one shall be subjected to arbitrary interference with his privacy, family, home or correspondence, nor to attacks upon his honor and reputation." The Organisation for Economic Co-operation and Development published its Privacy Guidelines in 1980. The European Union's 1995 Data Protection Directive guides privacy protection in Europe. The 2004 Privacy Framework by the Asia-Pacific Economic Cooperation is a privacy protection agreement for the members of that organization.

In the 1960s people began to consider how changes in technology were bringing changes in the concept of privacy. Vance Packard's The Naked Society was a popular book on privacy from that era and led discourse on privacy at that time.

PRIVACY LAW

Privacy law is the area of law concerning the protecting and preserving of privacy rights of individuals. While there is no universally accepted privacy law among all countries, some organizations promote certain concepts be enforced by individual countries.

For example, the Universal Declaration of Human Rights, Article 12, states:

No one shall be subjected to arbitrary interference with his privacy, family, home or correspondence, nor to attacks upon his honor and reputation. Everyone has the right to the protection of the law against such interference or attacks.

India and Privacy Laws

Indian privacy laws have been interpreted by the Indian Supreme Court in Article 21 of the Indian Constitution.

Cyberspace laws of India are not specified clearly. There is no such system that can easily track such practitioners in cyber world. However, nowadays demand to ensure the need of such laws has been significantly increased in India.

In 2015, Modi Government of India proposed dream project known as **"Digital India"**, in that context they should formed strong framework against phishing and internet crimes. Specialized training, modern equipment, awareness among population, ethical education for handling digital information and strict laws are necessary steps along with the expansion of digitalization in India.

Privacy in clinical Practice

Privacy is a fundamental right of every patient visited to clinician. The patient what discloses with doctor in either personal data, information, about sexual life, etc. should be kept confidential by him. It is doctor's moral responsibility to respect privacy of patient as individual. This should be cautiously considered while examining female patients. It is mandatory that there should be any female relative or nurse while attending female patient.

6

Whistleblower

LEARNING OBJECTIVES

After reading this chapter student should:
- Be able to define whistleblower and explain this concept in details
- Know about historical aspects of whistleblower
- Understand importance of whistleblower from the viewpoint of medical students
- Issue listed under whistleblower

INTRODUCTION

A **whistleblower** (**whistle-blower** or **whistle blower**) is a person who voluntarily discloses any kind of information or activity that is illegal, dishonest, or not correct within an organization that is either private or public.

Those who become whistleblowers can choose to bring information or allegations to surface either internally or externally. Internally, a whistleblower can bring his/her accusations to attention to other people within the accused organization. Externally, a whistleblower can bring allegations to light by contacting a third party outside of an accused organization. He/she can reach out to the media, government, law enforcement, or those who are concerned. whistleblowers also face stiff reprisal/retaliation from those whom are accused or alleged of wrongdoing. Third party groups like Wikileaks and others offer protection to whistleblowers, but that protection can only go so far. Whistleblowers face legal action,

33

criminal charges, social stigma, and termination from any position, office, or job.

Whistleblowers may be classified into: **Public and private.** However, whistleblowing in the public sector organization is more likely to result in federal felony charges and imprisonment. A whistleblower who chooses to accuse a private sector organization or agency is more likely to face termination and legal and civil charges.

Whistleblowing is not a new phenomenon. In fact it is thousands of years old. However, the decision and action has become far more complicated with recent advancements in technology and communication.

Origin of term

The term whistleblower arises from the whistle a referee uses to indicate an illegal or foul play. US civic activist Ralph Nader coined the phrase in the early 1970s to avoid the negative connotations found in other words such as "informers" and "snitches".

The definition of ethics is the moral principles that govern a person's or group's behavior. When it comes to whistleblowing most individuals perceive it as ethically wrong. Somewhat along the lines of tattle-telling or betraying loyalty, however what if by blowing the whistle a person saved the lives of multiple individuals? The ethical implications of whistleblowing can be negative as well as positive. However, sometimes employees may blow the whistle as an act of revenge.

Robert A. Larmer describes the standard view of whistleblowing in the Journal of Business Ethics by explaining that an employee possesses prima facie (based on the first impression; accepted as correct until proved otherwise) duties of loyalty and confidentiality to their employers and that whistleblowing cannot be justified except on the basis of a higher duty to the public good.

It is important to recognize that in any relationship which demands loyalty, the relationship works both ways and involves mutual enrichment.

MEDICAL STUDENTS AND WHISTLEBLOWING

This is an important concern with first-year medical students. As these are new students, certain important issues like ragging, college environment, hostel facilities, food quality in mess, hygiene in mess, stress, loneliness among students, teaching assessment, etc. can be collected under whistleblowing.

This information can be collected in systemic approach using of mentor schedule. Each trained mentor can carefully collects the information from students. This information will helpful in future planning and benefits for students. **Regular student counseling** and **mentorship programme implementation** can smoothly regulates medical students and decreases unnecessary stress over them.

As student whistleblowers the medical teachers should carefully handle the inputs obtained from students. The information which is collected from students should be confirmed before every action or implementation. Sometimes students may provide input such information that intentionally can trouble to other students.

It is the duty of every medical teacher to be producing promising environment to students.

The following is the list of issues cover under whistleblower expected from medical students.

1. Ragging
2. Understanding of subjects
3. Problems in hostel
4. College environment
5. Hostel facilities
6. Food quality in mess
7. Hygiene issue
8. Stress
9. Loneliness
10. Teaching assessment
11. Examination phobia
12. Interpersonal matter

7

Biocentrism

LEARNING OBJECTIVES

After reading this chapter student should:
- Be able to define biocentrism and zoocentrism
- Know about basic pillars of biocentrism
- Historical aspects of biocentrism
- Know about biocentrism in law
- Understand concept of relationship of biocentrism and religion
- Know about limitations of biocentrism

INTRODUCTION

Biocentrism (from Greek βίος (*bios*), "life" and κέντρον (*kentron*), "center"): Biocentrism is a concept that describes inherent value to every living thing with an objective to preserve environment, biodiversity and animal rights.

While the term **zoocentrism** limits inherent value specifically to animals.

Biocentrism deals with ethics of the relationship between humans and nature. It simply states that nature is not property of human but human is only part of that ecosystem. As higher species it is our responsibility to maintain regulations and to preserve our ecosystem for future.

PILLARS OF BIOCENTRISM

Following are four important pillars of Biocentrism.
1. Humans and all other species are members of our ecosystem.

2. All species are part of a system of interdependence.
3. All living organisms pursue their own "good" in their own ways.
4. Human beings are not inherently superior to other living things.

Relationship with Animals and Environment

In terms of ethical point of view and clarity, biocentrism and egocentrism are two different concepts. Biocentrism is based on concepts of ethics of individualism while ecocentrism provides moral priority to species rather than individual approach.

Biocentrism is based on ethical approach while ecocentrism is based on holistic approach.

HISTORY AND DEVELOPMENT

Biocentrism is quite differenst from traditional ethical thinking. Traditional ethical thinking is based on strict rules and regulations while biocentrism is based on attitude and character.

Traditional ethics provides priority to humankind while biocentrism provides priority to nature.

Biocentric ethics mainly includes Albert Schweitzer's ethics of "Reverence for Life", Peter Singer's ethics of Animal Liberation and Paul Taylor's (philosopher) ethics of biocentric egalitarianism.

Albert Schweitzer's "reverence for life" principle was a precursor of modern biocentric ethics.

In contrast with traditional ethics, the ethics of "reverence for life" denies any distinction between "high and low" or "valuable and less valuable" life forms, dismissing such categorization as arbitrary and subjective. Conventional ethics concerned itself exclusively with human beings, that is to say, morality applied only to interpersonal relationships, whereas Schweitzer's ethical philosophy introduced a "depth, energy, and function that differ[s] from the ethics that merely involved humans." "Reverence for life" was a "new ethics, because it is not only an extension of ethics, but also a transformation of the nature of ethics".

Similarly, Peter Singer argues that non-human animals deserve the same equality of consideration that we extend to human beings.

His argument is as follows:

1. Membership in the species *Homo sapiens* is the only criterion of moral importance that includes all humans and excludes all non-humans.

2. Using membership in the species *Homo sapiens* as a criterion of moral importance is completely arbitrary.

3. Of the remaining criteria we might consider, only sentience is a plausible criterion of moral importance.

4. Using sentience as a criterion of moral importance entails that we extend the same basic moral consideration (i.e. "basic principle of equality") to other sentient creatures that we do to human beings.

5. Therefore, we ought to extend to animals the same equality of consideration that we extend to human beings.

Biocentrism is most commonly associated with the work of Paul Taylor, especially his book *Respect for Nature: A Theory of Environmental Ethics* (1986). Taylor maintains that biocentrism is an "attitude of respect for nature", whereby one attempts to make an effort to live one's life in a way that respects the welfare and inherent worth of all living creatures.

Taylor states that:

1. Humans are members of a community of life along with all other species, and on equal terms.

2. This community consists of a system of interdependence between all members, both physically, and in terms of relationships with other species.

3. Every organism is a "teleological centre of life", that is, each organism has a purpose and a reason for being, which is inherently "good" or "valuable."

4. Humans are not inherently superior to other species.

In 1859, Charles Darwin published his book *On the Origin of Species*. This publication sparked the beginning of biocentrist views by introducing evolution and "its removal of humans from their supernatural origins and placement into the framework of natural laws".

The work of Aldo Leopold has also been associated with biocentrism.

The essay *The Land Ethic* in Leopold's book *Sand County Almanac* (1949) points out that although throughout history women and slaves have been considered property, all people have now been granted rights and freedoms. Leopold notes that today land is still considered property as people once were. He asserts that ethics should be extended to the land as "an evolutionary possibility and an ecological necessity". He argues that while people's instincts encourage them to compete with others, their ethics encourage them to co-operate with others. He suggests that "the land ethic simply enlarges the boundaries of the community to include soils, waters, plants, and animals, or collectively: the land". In a sense this attitude would encourage humans to co-operate with the land rather than compete with it.

Outside of formal philosophical works biocentric thought is common among pre-colonial tribal peoples who knew no world other than the natural world.

BIOCENTRISM IN LAW

The values that promote biocentrism for convenience are framed in terms of law.

Nowadays majority, countries in worldwide adopted laws concern with nature protection issue and biocentrism. The purpose of these laws are to prevent further degradation of nature and save our beautiful earth from distraction. The first country to include rights of nature in its constitution is Ecuador (See 2008 Constitution of Ecuador). Article 71 states that nature "has the right to integral respect for its existence and for the maintenance and regeneration of its life cycles, structure, functions and evolutionary processes".

There are various movements, NGOs are working over this issue in India and worldwide. The fear of pollution, damage of ozone layer, population exposure and consequent pollution, water crisis, loss of greenery, etc. are major concerns facing by us in twenty-first century.

To save our beautiful planet, it is our moral responsibility to adopt these ethical principles in our day to day life.

BIOCENTRISM AND RELIGION

Islam

In Islam, biocentric ethics stem from the belief that all of creation belongs to Allah (God), not humans, and to assume that non-human animals and plants exist merely to benefit humankind leads to environmental destruction and misuse. As all living organisms exist to praise God, human destruction of other living things prevents the earth's natural and subtle means of praising God. The Quran acknowledges that humans are not the only important creature and emphasizes a respect for nature. Muhammad was once asked whether there would be a reward for those who show charity to nature and animals, to which he replied, "for charity shown to each creature with a wet heart [i.e. alive], there is a reward."

Hinduism

Hinduism contains many elements of biocentrism. In Hinduism, humans have no special authority over other creatures, and all living things have souls ('atman'). Brahman (God) is the "efficient cause" and Prakrti (nature), is the "material cause" of the universe. However, Brahman and Prakrti are not considered truly divided: "They are one in the same, or perhaps better stated, they are the one in the many and the many in the one." However, while Hinduism does not give the same direct authority over nature that the Judeo-Christian God grants, they are subject to a "higher and more authoritative responsiblity for creation." The most important aspect of this is the doctrine of Ahimsa (non-violence). The essential aspect of this doctrine is the belief that the Supreme Being incarnates into the forms of various species.

The Hindu belief in samsāra (the cycle of life, death and rebirth) encompasses reincarnation into non-human forms. It is believed that one lives 84,000 lifetimes before one becomes a human. Each species is in this process of samsara until one attains moksha (liberation).

Another doctrinal source for the equal treatment of all life is found in the Rigveda. The Rigveda states that trees and plants possess divine healing properties. It is still popularly believed that every tree has a Vriksa-devata (a tree deity). Trees are ritually worshiped through prayer, offerings, and the sacred thread ceremony. The Vriksa-devata worshiped as manifestations of the divine. Tree planting is considered a religious duty.

Jainism

The Jaina tradition exists in tandem with Hinduism and shares many of its biocentric elements. **" Live and let live"** is the basic philosophy adopted by Jainism.

Parmodharam, Ahimsa (non-violence), the central teaching of Jainism, means more than not hurting other humans. It means intending not to cause physical, mental or spiritual harm to any part of nature. In the words of Mahavira: 'You are that which you wish to harm.' Compassion is a pillar of non-violence. Jainism encourages people to practice an attitude of compassion towards all life.

The principle of **interdependence** is also very important in Jainism. This states that all of nature is bound together, and that "if one does not care for nature, one does not care for oneself.".

Another essential Jain teaching is **self-restraint.**

Jainism discourages wasting the gifts of nature, and encourages its practitioners to reduce their needs as far as possible.

Gandhi, a great proponent of Jainism, once stated "There is enough in this world for human needs, but not for human wants."

Buddhism

In the Buddha's teachings encourage people "to live simply, to cherish tranquility, to appreciate the natural cycle of life." Buddhism emphasizes that everything in the universe affects everything else. "Nature is an ecosystem in which trees affect climate, the soil, and the animals, just as the climate affects the trees, the soil, the animals and so on. The ocean, the sky, the air are all interrelated, and interdependent—water is life and air is life."

Although this holistic approach is more ecocentric than biocentric, it is also biocentric, as it maintains that all living things are important and that humans are not above other creatures or nature. Buddhism teaches that "once we treat nature as our friend, to cherish it, then we can see the need to change from the attitude of dominating nature to an attitude of working with nature—we are an intrinsic part of all existence rather than seeing ourselves as in control of it."

CRITICISM AND BIOCENTRISM

There are a number of reasons or factors to criticize biocentrism concept. These can be listed as follows:

1. Too much importance is given to individual rather than group: In biocentrism whole importance is given to nature and each individual living cell. This leads human species back in action and be sensible with rules and regulations while exploiting the nature or damages to earth.

2. Biocentrism may act as an anti-human paradigm: Some authors felt biocentrism acts as an anti-human paradigm. By doing so these thought that human will act as inferior to others.

3. Biocentrism neglects ecosystem ethics: **Rule of survival** is always followed to maintain the balance of life in ecosystem. According to rule of survival one higher living species may damage to other lower living species to maintain his own survival. This is acceptable fact in ecosystem principles, which is not agreed in Biocentrism.

4. Biocentrism put human below the nature rather other theories accept human as higher power.

8

Human Decomposition

LEARNING OBJECTIVES

After reading this chapter student should:
• Be able to define cadaver and human decomposition
• Understand stages of decomposition
• Know about historical aspects of decomposition
• Know about body snatching events in ancient time

INTRODUCTION

A **cadaver**, also called a **corpse** in medical literature and legal usage or when intended for dissection, is a deceased human body.

STAGES OF DECOMPOSITION

1. **Autolysis (Self-digestion):** It is a first stage during which the body's cells are destroyed through the action of their own digestive enzymes. However, these enzymes are released into the cells because of active processes ceasing in the cells, not as an active process. In other words, though autolysis resembles the active process of digestion of nutrients by live cells, the dead cells are not actively digesting themselves as is often claimed in popular literature and as the synonym *self-digestion* of autolysis seems to imply. As a result of autolysis, liquid is created that gets between the layers of skin and makes the skin peel off. During this stage, flies start to lay eggs in the openings of the body: eyes, nostrils, mouth, ears, open wounds, and other orifices.

Hatched larvae (maggots) of blowflies, subsequently get under the skin and start to eat the body.

2. **Bloating:** It is a second stage in which bacteria in the gut begin to break down the tissues of the body, releasing gas that accumulates in the intestines, which becomes trapped because of the early collapse of the small intestine. This bloating occurs largely in the abdomen, and sometimes in the mouth and genitals. The tongue may swell. This usually happens in about the second week of decomposition. Gas accumulation and bloating will continue until the body is decomposed sufficiently for the gas to escape.

3. **Putrefaction:** It is the last and longest stage. Putrefaction is where the larger structures of the body break down, and tissues liquefy. The digestive organs, the brain, and lungs are the first to disintegrate. Under normal conditions, the organs are unidentifiable after three weeks. The muscles can be eaten by bacteria or devoured by animals. Eventually, sometimes after several years, all that remains is the skeleton.

HISTORY

Greek physician **Herophilus** known as the **"father of anatomy"**, lived in 300 BC in Alexandria, Egypt.

He was the first physician who dissected human body for the first time for academic purpose. The tradition of dissecting criminals was carried up into the eighteenth and nineteenth centuries when anatomy schools became popular in England and Scotland. At that time, a greater percentage of Christians believed in the literal raising from the dead. However, wrong believes such that souls of dissected bodies never go to heaven and such religious concepts was major obstacle in the process of body donation for medical schools.

Criminals who were executed for their crimes were used as the first cadavers. The demand for cadavers increased when the number of criminals being executed decreased. Since corpses were in such high demand, it became commonplace to steal bodies from graves in order to keep the market supplied.

The methods of preserving cadavers have changed over the last 200 years. At that time, cadavers had to be used immediately because there were no adequate methods to keep the body from quickly decaying. Preservation was needed in order to carry out classes and lessons about the human body. **Glutaraldehyde** was the first main chemical used for embalming and preserving the body although it leaves a yellow stain in the tissues, which can interfere with observation and research and thus interferes with anatomy teaching.

Formaldehyde is the chemical that is used as the main embalming chemical now. It is a colorless solution that maintains the tissue in its life-like texture and can keep the body well preserved for an extended period.

BODY SNATCHING

Anatomy schools began to steal bodies from graves. While "grave robbers" were technically people who stole jewelry from the deceased, some respected anatomy instructors dug up bodies themselves. The anatomist Thomas Sewall, who later became the personal physician for three US presidents, was convicted in 1818 of digging up a corpse for dissection.

Anatomists would even dissect members of their own family. William Harvey, the man famous for discovering the circulatory system, was so dedicated that he dissected his father and sister. From 1827 to 1828 in Scotland, murders were carried out, so that the bodies could be sold to medical schools for cash. These were known as the West Port murders. The Anatomy Act of 1832 was formed and passed because of the murders. H. H. Holmes, a noted serial killer in Chicago, Illinois, USA, sold the skeletons of some of his victims to medical schools.

By 1828 anatomists were paying others to do the digging. At that time, London Anatomy Schools employed ten full-time body snatchers and about 200 part-time workers during the dissection season. This period ran from October to May, when the winter cold slowed down the decomposition of the bodies. A crew of six or seven could dig up about 310 bodies.

The poor were most vulnerable, because they could not afford coffins to keep the body snatchers out.

Disposing of the dissected body was difficult, and rumors have appeared about how anatomists might have managed.

One possibility was secretly burying the remains behind their school. Another rumored possibility was that they gave the bodies to zoo-keepers, as feed for carnivorous animals or burial beneath elephant grazing pens, or fed the bodies to vultures kept specifically for this purpose.

Stories appeared of people murdering for the money they could make off cadaver sales.

Two of the most famous are that of Burke and Hare, and that of Bishop, May, and Williams.

- *Burke and Hare*—Burke and Hare ran a boarding house. When one of their tenants died, they brought him to Robert Knox's anatomy classroom in Edinburgh where they were paid seven pounds for the body. Realizing the possible profit, they murdered 16 people by asphyxiation over the next year and sold their bodies to Knox. They were eventually caught when a tenant returned to her bed only to encounter a corpse. Hare testified against Burke in exchange for amnesty and Burke was found guilty, hanged, and publicly dissected.

- **London Burkers, Bishop, May and Williams** — These body snatchers also killed three boys, ages 10, 11 and 14 years old. The anatomist that they sold the cadavers to was suspicious. To delay their departure the anatomist said he needed to break a 50-pound note. He sent the police who arrested the men. In Bishop's confession he stated, "I have followed the course of obtaining a livelihood as a body snatcher for 12 years, and have obtained and sold, I think from 500 to 1,000 bodies"

Nowadays we are very lucky that we receive sufficient bodies for dissection purpose in medical colleges in India. As medical student we should understand importance of these bodies. The credits go to various body donation activist programmes conducted by various institutions and increment of awareness among citizens.

9

Embalming

LEARNING OBJECTIVES

After reading this chapter student should:
• Be able to define and explain process of embalming
• Know about uses/indications of embalming
• Know about process of embalming
• Know about historical aspects of embalming
• Know about modern practices of embalming
• Understand concept of embalming and ethical approach

INTRODUCTION

Embalming is an art and science of preserving human body by specially treating them to prevent from decomposition and can be used for academic as well as nonacademic purposes.

When a corpse is buried, the body will decompose by the actions of anaerobic bacteria. In many countries, corpses buried in coffins are embalmed. An embalmer may prepare the corpse for a life-like appearance. Embalming fluid is then pumped into the body via a common carotid or femoral artery. This by rehydration process reduces decomposition and maintains structural stability.

There are controversial opinions worldwide over embalming practices. Most of the time embalming is done for research and dissection purposes in medical colleges. Sometimes it may be done for preserving body for some days due to delay in funeral process due to some reasons, etc. Religious faiths are the major obstacle in embalming practices in worldwide scenario. There

47

is need to change mindset of people. However, it is promising fact that nowadays there are dramatic changes in the attitude of people.

The bodies can be maintained for about 3–4 years by this process.

The three basic goals of embalming are **sanitization, presentation** and **preservation.** The sanitization means prevent these bodies from decomposition. The presentation means these bodies can be preserved for funeral process if delayed due to any social reason, etc. While preservation means maintain these bodies for research or teaching purpose.

The embalming is one of the most important necessary processes in maintainning bodies for dissection for 1–2 years in dissection hall and handle by medical students.

HISTORY

The embalming has a long traditional, societal and cultural history.

The Chinchorro culture in the Atacama desert of present day Chile and Peru are among the earliest cultures known to have performed artificial mummification as early as 5000–6000 BC. Perhaps the ancient culture that had developed embalming to the greatest extent was that of Egypt, where as early as the first dynasty (3200 BC) specialized priests were in charge of embalming and mummification. The ancient Egyptians believed that preservation of the mummy empowered the soul after death, the latter of which would return to the preserved corpse.

The first attempt to inject the vascular system were made by Alessandro Giliani of Persiceto, who died in 1326.

In the 19th and early 20th centuries arsenic was frequently used as an embalming fluid but has since been supplanted by other more effective and less toxic chemicals.

Embalming is different from taxidermy. Embalming preserves the human body intact, whereas taxidermy is the recreation of an animal's form often using only the creature's skin mounted on an anatomical form.

Modern embalming is most often performed to ensure a better presentation of the deceased for viewing by friends and relatives—as everything else being equal, an embalmed body will look better than one that is unembalmed and putrefying. In the United Kingdom, where open casket funerals are extremely rare, embalming is still used in many funeral homes.

MODERN PRACTICES

The actual embalming process usually involves four parts:

1. **Arterial embalming,** which involves the injection of embalming chemicals into the blood vessels, usually via the right common carotid artery. Blood and interstitial fluids are displaced by this injection and, along with excess arterial solution, are expelled from the right jugular vein and collectively referred to as drainage. The embalming solution is injected with a centrifugal pump and the embalmer massages the body to break up circulatory clots as to ensure the proper distribution of the embalming fluid. This process of raising vessels with injection and drainage from a solitary location is known as a single-point injection.

2. **Cavity embalming** refers to the replacement of internal fluids inside body cavities with embalming chemicals via the use of anaspirator and trocar.

3. **Hypodermic embalming** is a supplemental method which refers to the injection of embalming chemicals into tissue with a hypodermic needle and syringe, which is generally used as needed on a case by case basis to treat areas where arterial fluid has not been successfully distributed during the main arterial injection.

4. **Surface embalming,** another supplemental method, utilizes embalming chemicals to preserve and restore areas directly on the skin's surface and other superficial areas as well as areas of damage such as from accident, decomposition, cancerous growth or skin donation.

A typical embalming takes several hours to complete.

Chemicals

Typical embalming fluid contains a mixture of formaldehyde, glutaraldehyde, ethanol, humectants, and wetting agents and other solvents that can be used. The formaldehyde content generally ranges from 5 to 35 percent and the ethanol content may range from 9 to 56 percent.

Specialist embalming

Badly decomposing bodies, trauma cases, frozen or drowned bodies, and those to be transported over long distances also require special treatment beyond that for the "normal" case. The restoration of bodies and features damaged by accident or disease is commonly called restorative art or demi-surgery and all qualified embalmers have some degree of training and practice in it. For such cases, the benefit of embalming is startlingly apparent.

Embalming autopsy cases differs from standard embalming because the nature of the post-mortem examination irrevocably disrupts the circulatory system, due to the removal of the organs and viscera. In these cases, a six-point injection is made through the two iliac or femoral arteries, subclavian or axillary vessels, and common carotids, with the viscera treated separately with cavity fluid or a special embalming powder in a viscera bag, "shake and bake".

Long-term preservation requires different techniques, such as using stronger preservative chemicals and multiple injection sites to ensure thorough saturation of body tissues.

EMBALMING AND ETHICS

The decision of embalming is generally taken by close relatives of the person after his death. In very exceptional cases the person already declares will to use his body for research purpose or dissection purpose in medical institutions after his death. Though there is no clear guidelines regarding embalming and its applications, but due to various movements like body donation scheme by medical institutions for increasing awareness and will of people there is noted positive results. However, in India majority of the bodies which were used for dissection purpose were obtained as unclaimed bodies collected by police. Nowadays this scenario is changing.

10

Eugenics

LEARNING OBJECTIVES

After reading this chapter student should:
• Be able to define and explain eugenics.
• Know about historical aspects and practices of eugenics in world and India
• Understand concept of unfit vs. fit individuals in eugenics
• Know about "compulsory sterilization" campaign
• Understand issues concerned with eugenics and ethical aspects.

INTRODUCTION

Societal movement is born for improved and beneficiary genetic features of future human population using selective breeding and sterilization is known as **eugenics.**

Eugenics was practised in the United States many years before eugenics programs in Nazi Germany and US programs provided much of the inspiration for the latter.

Stefan Kühl has documented the consensus between Nazi race policies and those of eugenicists in other countries, including the United States, and points out that eugenicists understood Nazi policies and measures as the realization of their goals and demands.

In early 20th century this was considered a method for preserving and improving the dominant groups in the society.

HISTORICAL ASPECTS AND PRACTICES OF EUGENICS IN WORLD AND INDIA

The American eugenics movement was rooted in the biological determinist ideas of Sir Francis Galton, which originated in the 1880s. Galton studied the upper classes of Britain, and arrived at the conclusion that their social positions were due to a superior genetic makeup. Early proponents of eugenics believed that, through selective breeding, the human species should direct its own evolution. They tended to believe in the genetic superiority of Nordic, Germanic and Anglo-Saxon peoples; supported strict immigration and anti-miscegenation laws; and supported the forcible sterilization of the poor, disabled and "immoral".

In 1906, J H Kellogg provided funding to help found the Race Betterment Foundation in Battle Creek, Michigan. The Eugenics Record Office (ERO) was founded in Cold Spring Harbor, New York in 1911 by the renowned biologist Charles B. Davenport, using money from both the Harriman railroad fortune and the Carnegie Institution. As late as the 1920s, the ERO was one of the leading organizations in the American eugenics movement.

Eugenics was widely accepted in the US academic community.

Public acceptance in the US was the reason of eugenic legislation to be passed. Almost 19 million people attended the Panama-Pacific International Exposition in San Francisco, open for 10 months from February 20 to December 4, 1915.

IMMIGRATION RESTRICTIONS

The Immigration Restriction League was the first American entity associated officially with eugenics. Founded in 1894 by three recent Harvard University graduates, the League sought to bar what it considered inferior races from entering America and diluting what it saw as the superior American racial stock (upper class Northerners of Anglo-Saxon heritage). They felt that social and sexual involvement with these less-evolved and less-civilized races would pose a biological threat to the American population.

With the passage of the Immigration Act of 1924, eugenicists for the first time played an important role in the Congressional debate as expert advisers on the threat of "inferior stock" from eastern and southern Europe.

Unfit vs. Fit Individuals

Both class and race factored into eugenic definitions of "fit" and "unfit." By using intelligence testing, American eugenicists asserted that social mobility was indicative of one's genetic fitness. This reaffirmed the existing class and racial hierarchies and explained why the upper-to-middle class was predominately white. Middle-to-upper class status was a marker of "superior strains." In contrast, eugenicists believed poverty to be a characteristic of genetic inferiority, which meant that that those deemed "unfit" were predominately of the lower classes.

Because class status designated some more fit than others, eugenicists treated upper and lower class women differently. Positive eugenicists, who promoted procreation among the fittest in society, encouraged middle class women to bear more children. Between 1900 and 1960, Eugenicists appealed to middle class white women to become more "family minded," and to help better the race. To this end, eugenicists often denied middle and upper class women sterilization and birth control.

COMPULSORY STERILIZATION

In 1907, Indiana passed the first eugenics-based compulsory sterilization law in the world.

Thirty US states would soon follow their lead. Although the law was overturned by the Indiana Supreme Court in 1921, the US Supreme Court upheld the constitutionality of a Virginia law allowing for the compulsory sterilization of patients of state mental institutions in 1927.

The most significant era of eugenic sterilization was between 1907 and 1963, when over 64,000 individuals were forcibly sterilized under eugenic legislation alone in the United States.

Beginning around 1930, there was a steady increase in the percentage of women sterilized, and in a few states only young women were sterilized. From 1930 to the 1960s, sterilizations were performed on many more institutionalized women than men. By 1961, 61 percent of the 62,162 total eugenic sterilizations in the United States were performed on women.

Men and women were compulsorily sterilized for legally different reasons. Men were specially sterilized to treat their aggression and to eliminate their criminal tendency, while women were specially sterilized to control the results of their will and sexuality. Since women bore children, eugenicists held women more accountable than men for the reproduction of the less "desirable" members of society. Eugenicists therefore predominately targeted women in their efforts to regulate the birth rate, to "protect" white racial health, and weed out the "defectives" of society.

Although the sterilizations were not explicitly motivated by eugenics, the sterilizations were similar to the eugenics movement because they were done without the patients' consent.

EUGENICS AND ETHICAL ASPECTS

Eugenics is ideally based on concept beneficiary for future human population; however, from ethical point of view is it justifiable? Dominant always rules the world is the law of nature. Ethics always based on equality and justice either the person is rich or poor.

Is eugenics can implement through governance? Is it justice for lower strata of population? What for autonomy of individual? If cloning is the mantra of future world for human benefits then what is meant for morals?

The future world experiments like SENS and advancement in medical care leading increment in age of human. The human is travelling towards immortality. Herewith today we are on the mode of time asking for future. Nanotechnology and its advancements, techno-human population, virtual life experience based new generation; definitely it is time to rethink.

Proposed fundamentals of medical bioethics by various researchers and their debates are today's need.

11

Euthanasia

LEARNING OBJECTIVES

After reading this chapter student should:
- Be able to define and explain euthanasia
- Know about practices of euthanasia in worldwide scenario
- Understand classification of euthanasia
- Know about euthanasia in India
- Know about "Aruna Shanbaug case"
- Understand implications of medical bioethics in euthanasia

INTRODUCTION

Euthanasia or mercy killing is one of the most controversial issues in medical bioethics worldwide scenario. Netherland was the first country to legalize euthanasia in 2008. While some countries have accepted euthanasia as a part of medical practice, the debate over it still continues.

In early days euthanasia was practiced to get rid of "inferior" as well as the old and deliberated population as a way of promoting a healthy and genetically "superior" and young population for betterment purposes.

In India euthanasia is traditionally practiced in some part of southern districts of Tamil Nadu.

PRACTICES OF EUTHANASIA IN WORLD

By 1925 the Eugenics Records Office was distributing standardized forms for judging eugenically fit families, which were used in contests in several US states.

After the **eugenics movement** was well established in the **United States**, it spreads to **Germany.**

California eugenicists started producing literature which promoting eugenics and sterilization and sending it overseas to German medical professionals. By 1933, California had subjected more people to forceful sterilization than all other US states combined. The forced sterilization program was formed by the Nazis was partly inspired by California's thinking and based on literature.

The Rockefeller Foundation helped develop and fund to number of German eugenics programs, including the one that Josef Mengele worked in before he went to Auschwitz.

In 1934, where more than 5,000 people per month were being forcibly sterilized, the California eugenics activist C. M. Goethe write:

"You will be interested to know that your work has played a powerful part in shaping the opinions of the group of intellectuals who are behind Hitler in this epoch-making program. Everywhere I sensed that their opinions have been tremendously stimulated by American thought . . . I want you, my dear friend, to carry this thought with you for the rest of your life, that you have really jolted into action a great government of 60 million people."

Eugenics activist Harry H. Laughlin often bragged that his Model Eugenic Sterilization laws had been implemented in 1935 Nuremberg racial hygiene laws. In 1936, Laughlin was invited to an award ceremony at Heidelberg University in Germany (scheduled on the anniversary of Hitler's 1934 purge of Jews from the Heidelberg faculty), to receive an honorary doctorate for his work on the "science of racial cleansing". Due to financial limitations, Laughlin was unable to attend the ceremony and had to pick it up from the Rockefeller Institute.

After 1945, however, historians started to attempt to portray the US eugenics movement as distinct and distant from Nazi eugenics. Jon Entine wrote that eugenics simply means "good genes" and using it as synonym for genocide is an "all-too-common distortion of the social history of genetics policy in the United States." According to Entine, eugenics developed out of the Progressive Era and not "Hitler's twisted Final Solution."

Classification of Euthanasia

Euthanasia can be simply classified into four major groups, viz. voluntary euthanasia, non-voluntary euthanasia, involuntary euthanasia and passive euthanasia.

1. **Voluntary euthanasia:** In voluntary euthanasia person asks for killing voluntarily with cautiously and willfully.

2. **Non-voluntary euthanasia:** In non-voluntary euthanasia person is not able to take decision. He may be either mentally unfit, in coma, younger baby, severe brain damage or mentally disturbed.

3. **Involuntary euthanasia:** Euthanasia is conducted without the patient consent.

4. **Passive euthanasia:** In passive euthanasia patient dies due to withholding of medical treatment like switch of life support measures, disconnect feeding tube, etc.

Euthanasia and India

Passive euthanasia is legally allowed in India.

On 7 March 2011 the Supreme Court of India legalized passive euthanasia by means of the withdrawal of life support to patients in a permanent vegetative state.

The decision was made as part of the verdict in a case involving Aruna Shanbaug, who had been in a Persistent Vegetative State (PVS) until her death in 2015.

In March 2011, the Supreme Court of India, passed a historic judgement-law permitting Passive Euthanasia in the country. This judgment was passed in wake of Pinki Virani's plea to the highest court in December 2009 under the Constitutional provision of "Next Friend". It is a milestone law which places the power of choice in the hands of the individual, over government, medical or religious control which sees all suffering as "destiny". The Supreme Court specified two irreversible conditions to permit Passive Euthanasia Law in its 2011 law: (I) The brain-dead for whom the ventilator can be switched off (II) Those in a Persistent Vegetative State (PVS) for whom the feed can be tapered out and pain-managing palliatives be added, according to laid-down international specifications.

The same judgement-law also asked for the scrapping of 309, the code which penalises those who survive suicide-attempts. In December 2014, Government of India declared its intention to do so.

However on 25 February 2014, a three-judge bench of Supreme Court of India had termed the judgment in Aruna Shanubauge case to be 'inconsistent in itself' and has referred the issue of euthanasia to its five-judge constitution bench.

On December 23, 2014, Government of India endorsed and re-validated the Passive Euthanasia judgement-law in a Press Release, after stating in the Rajya Sabha as follows: that The Honourable Supreme Court of India in its judgment dated 7.3.2011 [WP (Criminal) No. 115 of 2009], while dismissing the plea for mercy killing in a particular case, laid down comprehensive guidelines to process cases relating to passive euthanasia. Thereafter, the matter of mercy killing was examined in consultation with the Ministry of Law and Justice and it has been decided that since the Honourable Supreme Court has already laid down the guidelines, these should be followed and treated as law in such cases. At present, there is no proposal to enact legislation on this subject and the judgment of the Honourable Supreme Court is binding on all.

The high court rejected active euthanasia by means of lethal injection.

Active euthanasia, including the administration of lethal compounds for the purpose of ending life, is still illegal in India, and in most countries.

Aruna Shanbaug Case

Aruna Shanbaug was a nurse working at the King Edward Memorial Hospital, Parel, Mumbai. On 27 November 1973 she was strangled and sodomized by a sweeper. During the attack she was strangled with a chain, and the deprivation of oxygen has left her in a vegetative state ever since. She has been treated at KEM since the incident and is kept alive by feeding tube. On behalf of Aruna, her friend Pinki Virani, a social activist, filed a petition in the Supreme Court arguing that the "continued existence of Aruna is in violation of her right to live in dignity". The Supreme Court made its decision on 7 March 2011. The court rejected the plea to discontinue Aruna's life support but issued a set of broad guidelines legalising passive euthanasia in India. The Supreme Court's decision to reject the discontinuation of Aruna's life support was based on the fact that the hospital staff who treat and take care of her did not support euthanizing her. She died from pneumonia on 18 May 2015, after being in a coma for 42 years.

While rejecting Pinki Virani's plea for Aruna Shanbaug's euthanasia, the court laid out guidelines for passive euthanasia.

According to these guidelines, passive euthanasia involves the withdrawing of treatment or food that would allow the patient to live.

Forms of active euthanasia, including the administration of lethal compounds, legal in a number of nations and jurisdictions including Belgium and the Netherlands, as well as the US states of Washington and Oregon, are still illegal in India.

Elsewhere in the world active euthanasia is almost always illegal. The legal status of passive euthanasia, on the other hand, including the withdrawal of nutrition or water, varies across the nations of the world. As India had no law about euthanasia, the Supreme Court's guidelines are law until and unless Parliament passes legislation.

The following guidelines were laid down :

1. A decision has to be taken to discontinue life support either by the parents or the spouse or other close relatives, or in the absence of any of them, such a decision can be taken even by a person or a body of persons acting as a next friend. It can also be taken by the doctors attending the patient. However, the decision should be taken bona fide in the best interest of the patient.

2. Even if a decision is taken by the near relatives or doctors or next friend to withdraw life support, such a decision requires approval from the High Court concerned.

3. When such an application is filled the Chief Justice of the High Court should forthwith constitute a Bench of at least two Judges who should decide to grant approval or not. A committee of three reputed doctors to be nominated by the Bench, who will give report regarding the condition of the

patient. Before giving the verdict a notice regarding the report should be given to the close relatives and the State. After hearing the parties, the High Court can give its verdict. Court has referred the issue to a constitution bench which shall be heard by a strength of at least five judges. Court observed:

In view of the inconsistent opinions rendered in Aruna Shanbaug (supra) and also considering the important question of law involved which needs to be reflected in the light of social, legal, medical and constitutional perspective, it becomes extremely important to have a clear enunciation of law. Thus, in our cogent opinion, the question of law involved requires careful consideration by a Constitution Bench of this Court for the benefit of humanity as a whole.

After the court ruling The Telegraph consulted with Muslim, Hindu, Jain and Christian religious leaders. Though generally against legalising euthanasia, Christians and the Jains thought passive euthanasia was acceptable under some circumstances.

Jains and Hindus have the traditional rituals Santhara and Prayopavesa respectively, wherein one can end one's life by starvation, when one feels their life is complete.

EUTHANASIA AND MEDICAL ETHICS

It is really a controversial issue. But on the basis of autonomy it is patient right or on the patient will, he can chose his treatment plan. But when patient is not in such state when he can decide, it is moral responsibility of his close relatives to decide what to finalize. Many countries agreed over this fact. However, this is very situational decision which doctors has to face. It is also clinician's responsibility to get justice to his patient.

12

Genetic Counseling

LEARNING OBJECTIVES

After reading this chapter student should:
- Be able to define and explain concept of genetic counseling
- Know about structure of genetic counseling
- Know about list of conditions of genetic counseling
- Understand concept of prenatal genetic counseling

INTRODUCTION

The National Society of Genetic Counselors (NSGC) officially defines genetic counseling as the understanding and adaptation to the medical, psychological and familial implications of genetic contributions to disease.

This process integrates:
- Interpretation of family and medical histories to assess the chance of disease occurrence or recurrence.
- Education about inheritance, testing, management, prevention, resources
- Counseling to promote informed choices and adaptation to the risk or condition.

Genetic counselor is an expert with skillful in translating the complex genomic medicine language into easy concepts and terms that can easily understand to patients. He can be from any streams of education either biology, nursing, psychology, societal work, medicine, etc. There are nationwide various associations that certify these counselors.

Genetic counselors act as coordinator between physicians and patients as well as genetic resource to physicians. Genetic counselors provide information and support to families who have members with birth defects or genetic disorders, and to families who may be at risk for a variety of inherited conditions. They identify families at risk, investigate the problems present in the family, interpret information about the disorder, analyze inheritance patterns and risks of recurrence, and review available genetic testing options with the family.

Genetic counselors are present at high risk or specialty prenatal clinics that offer prenatal diagnosis, pediatric care centers, and adult genetic centers. Genetic counseling can occur before conception (i.e. when one or two of the parents are carriers of a certain trait) through to adulthood (for adult onset genetic conditions, such as Huntington's disease or hereditary cancer syndromes).

PATIENTS

Any person may seek out genetic counseling for a condition they may have inherited from their biological parents.

A woman, if pregnant, may be referred for genetic counseling if a risk is discovered through prenatal testing (screening or diagnosis). Some clients are notified of having a higher individual risk for chromosomal abnormalities or birth defects. Testing enables women and couples to make a decision as to whether or not to continue with their pregnancy, and helps provide information that can be used to prepare for the birth of a child with medical issues.

A person may also undergo genetic counseling after the birth of a child with a genetic condition. In these instances, the genetic counselor explains the condition to the patient along with recurrence risks in the future children. In all cases of a positive family history for a condition, the genetic counselor can evaluate risks, recurrence and explain the condition itself.

COUNSELING SESSION STRUCTURE

The goals of genetic counseling are to increase understanding of genetic diseases, discuss disease management options, and explain the risks and benefits of testing. Counseling sessions focus on giving vital, unbiased information and non-directive assistance in the patient's decision-making process. Seymour Kessler, in 1979, first categorized sessions in five phases: an intake phase, an initial contact phase, the encounter phase, the summary phase, and a follow-up phase. The intake and follow-up phases occur outside of the actual counseling session. The initial contact phase is when the counselor and families meet and build rapport. The encounter phase includes dialogue between the counselor and the client about the nature of screening and diagnostic tests. The summary phase provides all the options and decisions available for the next step. If counselees wish to go ahead with testing, an appointment is organized and the genetic counselor acts as the person to communicate the results.

Reasons and Results

Families or individuals may choose to attend counseling or undergo prenatal testing for a number of reasons.

• Family history of a genetic condition or chromosome abnormality
• Molecular test for single gene disorder
• Increased maternal age (35 years and older)
• Increased paternal age (40 years and older)
• Abnormal maternal serum screening results or ultrasound findings
• Increased nuchal translucency measurements on ultrasound
• Strong family history of cancer
• Predictive testing for adult-onset conditions

Conditions

Many disorders cannot occur unless both the mother and father pass on their genes, such as cystic fibrosis. Some diseases can be inherited from one parent, such as Huntington disease, and DiGeorge syndrome. Other genetic disorders are the cause of an error or mutation occurring during the cell division process (e.g. trisomy). Testing can reveal conditions that are easily treatable as long as they are detected (Phenylketonuria or PKU). Genetic tests are available for a number of genetic conditions including but not limited to:

- Down syndrome
- Sickle-cell anemia
- Tay-Sachs disease
- Muscular dystrophy

Genetic Counselors as Support

Genetic alliance states that counselors provide supportive counseling to families, serve as patient advocates and refer individuals and families to community or state support services. They serve as educators and resource people for other healthcare professionals and for the general public. Many engage in research activities related to the field of medical genetics and genetic counseling. The field of genetic counseling is rapidly expanding and many counselors are taking on "non-traditional roles" which includes working for genetic companies and laboratories. When communicating increased risk, counselors anticipate the likely distress and prepare patients for the results. Counselors help clients cope with and adapt to the emotional, psychological, medical, social, and economic consequences of the test results.

Each individual considers his family needs, social setting, cultural background, and religious beliefs when interpreting his risk. Clients must evaluate their reasoning to continue with testing at all. Counselors are present to put all the possibilities in perspective and encourage clients to take time to think about their decision. When a risk is found, counselors frequently reassure parents that they were not responsible for the result. An informed choice without pressure or coercion is made when all relevant information has been given and understood.

Prenatal Genetic Counseling

If an initial noninvasive screening test reveals a risk to the baby, patients are encouraged to attend genetic counseling to learn about their options. Further prenatal investigation is beneficial and provides helpful details regarding the status of the fetus, contributing to the decision-making process. Decisions made by patients are affected by factors including timing, accuracy of information provided by tests, and risk and benefits of the tests. Counselors present a summary of all the options available.

Patients may accept the risk and have no future testing, proceed to diagnostic testing, or take further screening tests to refine the risk. Invasive diagnostic tests possess a small risk of miscarriage (1–2%) but provide more definitive results. While families seek direction and suggestions from the counselors, they are reassured that no right or wrong answer exists. When discussing possible choices, counselor discourse predominates and is characterized by examples of what some people might do. Discussion enables people to place the information and circumstances into the context of their own lives. Patients are given a decision-making framework they can use to situate themselves. Counselors focus on the importance of individual choice based on the experiences, morals, and viewpoints of the couple/individual/family. Testing is offered to provide a definitive answer regarding the presence of a certain genetic condition or chromosomal abnormality. There is often no therapy or treatment available for these conditions, and as such parents may choose to terminate the pregnancy.

Referral

After attending prenatal counseling, women have the option of accepting the risk revealed and having no further investigations during their pregnancy. They may choose to undergo noninvasive screening (e.g. ultrasound, triple screen, cell-free fetal DNA screening) or invasive diagnostic testing (amniocentesis or chorionic villus sampling).

After counseling for other hereditary conditions, the patient may be presented with the option of having genetic testing. In some circumstances no genetic testing is indicated, other times it may be useful to begin the testing process with an affected family member. The genetic counselor also reviews the advantages and disadvantages of genetic testing with the patient.

Attitudes toward Counseling

The plethora of information available can be overwhelming and counselors spend a large proportion of time clarifying details. Prenatal screening was first introduced nearly four decades ago, yet gaps still exist in public knowledge about the screening program. The general public is familiar with Down syndrome (trisomy 21), but is not aware of more uncommon conditions such as trisomy 18 (historically known as Edwards syndrome) and trisomy 13 (Patau syndrome). Clients are usually aware of diagnostic testing from friends, TV/press, or because of family history. No simple correlation has been found between the change in technology to the changes in values and beliefs towards genetic testing.

13

Organ Donation

LEARNING OBJECTIVES

After reading this chapter student should:
- Be able to define and explain concept of organ donation
- Be able to define allotransplantations, xenotransplantation, explicit consent and presumed consent
- Know about consent process in organ donation
- Know about Indian Organ Donation Act
- Know about "Tamil Nadu model of organ donation"
- Understand different religious views and organ donation
- Know some notable donators list

INTRODUCTION

Organ donation is defined as donation of biological tissue or an organ of the human body, from a living or dead person within specified time limit, to a living recipient in need of a transplantation.

Such transplantation procedure from human to human is known as **allotransplantations**.

The transfer of animal organs into human bodies is known as **xenotransplantation**.

Transplantation is based on the donor's medical and social history.

In global scenario, there is seen large gap between the numbers of registered donors compared to those awaiting organ donations.

CONSENT PROCESS

The consent process for organ donation is basically of two types, viz. explicit consent (opt-in system) and presumed consent (opt-out system).

Explicit consent consists of the donor giving direct consent through proper registration depending on the country. While the **presumed consent,** which does not need direct consent from the donor or the next of kin. Presumed consent assumes that donation would have been permitted by the potential donor if permission was pursued. Of possible donors an estimated twenty-five percent of families refuse to donate a loved one's organs.

In global survey study, the countries which use presumed consent having high numbers of transplants compared to who use explicit consent.

INDIA AND ORGAN DONATION

Indian government in 1994 introduced law "The Transplantation of Human Organs Act" **really brought significant changes in the organ donation and transplantation scene in India.** Corneal donation programme is having good success. Despite such law there have been stray instances of organ trade in India.

Tamil Nadu Model

Tamil Nadu is the leader in deceased organ donation in the country. This is possible due to combined effect of both government and private hospitals, NGOs and the State Health department. In the year 2000, through the efforts of an NGO, MOHAN Foundation state of Tamil Nadu started an organ sharing network between a few hospitals. In 2008, the Government of Tamil Nadu put together government orders laying down procedures and guidelines for deceased organ donation and transplantation in the state.

There are such different programs and efforts adopted by state ministries in India.

• Andhra Pradesh—Jeevandan programme
• Karnataka—Zonal Coordination Committee of Karnataka for Transplantation

- Kerala—Mrithasanjeevani—The Kerala Network for Organ Sharing
- Maharashtra—Zonal Transplant Coordination Center in Mumbai
- Tamil Nadu—Cadaver Transplant Programme

In the year 2012 besides Tamil Nadu other southern states to do deceased donation transplants more frequently. An online organ sharing registry for deceased donation and transplantation is used by the states of Tamil Nadu (www. tnos.org) and Kerala (www.knos.org.in). Both these registries have been developed, implemented and maintained by MOHAN Foundation.

Organ selling is legally banned in Asia. Numerous studies have documented that organ vendors have a poor *quality of life* (QOL) following kidney donation. However, a study done by Vemuru reddy *et al* shows a significant improvement in quality of life contrary to the earlier belief. Live related renal donors have a significant improvement in the QOL following renal donation using the WHO QOL BREF in a study done at the All India Institute of Medical Sciences from 2006 to 2008. The quality of life of the donor was poor when the graft was lost or the recipient died.

Religious Views and Organ Donation

All major religions accept organ donation in at least some form on either utilitarian ground (i.e. because of its life-saving capabilities) or deontological ground (e.g. the right of an individual believer to make his or her own decision). Most religions, among them the Roman Catholic Church, support organ donation on the ground that it constitutes an act of charity and provides a means of saving a life, consequently Pope Francis is an organ donor. One religious group, The Jesus Christians, became known as "The Kidney Cult" because more than half of its members had donated their kidneys altruistically. Jesus Christians claimed altruistic kidney donation is a great way to "Do unto others what they would want you to do unto them." Some religions placed some restrictions on the types of organs that may be donated and/ or on the means by which organs may be harvested and/or transplanted. For example, Jehovah's witnesses require that organs be drained of any blood due to their interpretation of the Hebrew Bible/Christian Old Testament as prohibiting blood transfusion, and Muslims require that the donors have provided written consent in advance. A few groups disfavor organ transplantation or donation; notably, these include Shinto and those who follow the customs of the Gypsies.

Judaism considers organ donation obligatory if it will save a life, as long as the donor is considered dead as defined by Jewish law. In both Judaism the majority view holds that organ donation is permitted in the case of irreversible cardiac rhythm cessation. In some more cases, rabbinic authorities believe that organ donation may be mandatory, whereas a minority opinion considers any donation of a live organ as forbidden.

SHORTAGE OF ORGAN DONATION

Currently more than 100,000 people are waiting for an organ transplant, yet there is a shortage of donors. Over the years people all over the world have stopped registering to be organ donors causing many people to die each year. The shortage is causing countries all over the world to go to drastic measures of getting donors. Such as, paying them for the said organs needed. Although, organs may only be taken from donors that have been declared dead (brain-dead). The shortage of organs have increased because of criteria among certain organs. For example, a kidney transplant would be less likely to fail if it was donated by young, healthy donors other than older donors who have had medical issues in their past. This is causing too much pressure amongst people to donate. More countries have been moving toward making everyone an organ donor unless they have a signed consent disregarding them from donating. People are even selling organs and causing black market sales with insufficient postoperative care to patients. Other than this health and safety issue, the organ shortage can be solved by paying people to donate. This leading to the ethical dispute of people saying "no give, no take." This stating that if they are willing to give then they should be first to receive if needed. Also stating that each person would receive points for every relative who signs a donor card as well as them. Without such techniques to help increase donors then the amount of organs for transplant patients will gradually and drastically decrease over time.

Some Notable Donators

Manikanta, a 22-year-old car driver, suffered a brain injury in road accident on March 3, 2015 in Vijayawada, India. His family decided to donate his vital organs to save 8 lives. By making this donation, it prevented perfectly functionable organs to die with the patient.

14

Religious Practices of Embalming

LEARNING OBJECTIVES

After reading this chapter student should:
• Know about religious practices of embalming
• Know list of notable embalming in history
• Understand values of ethics in embalming
• Know about implications of embalming

INTRODUCTION

Worldwide there are controversial opinions over embalming practices. Most of time embalming is done for research and dissection purpose in medical colleges. Sometimes it may be done for preserving body for some days due to delay in funeral process due to some reasons, etc. Religious faiths are the major obstacle in embalming practices in worldwide scenario. There is need to change mindset of people. However, it is promising fact that nowadays there are dramatic changes in attitude of people.

Following is the list of opinions concerned with various realigns and their routine process:

• Most branches of the Christian faith generally allow embalming. Some bodies within Eastern Orthodoxy profess strongly ban against embalming except when required by lawfully or other necessity, while others may discourage but do not prohibit it. In general the decision on embalming is one that is dictated by the personal preference of the family rather than a specific church policy.

- The Church of Jesus Christ of latter-day saints does not discourage or prohibit embalming. Often, due to the custom of church members dressing the deceased, embalming is given preference.

- Some Neopagans generally discourage embalming, believing it unnatural to disrupt the physical recycling of the body to the earth in the mistaken belief that embalmed bodies do not decompose. They encourage the use of green graveyards, where the body is placed in a biodegradable casket and buried under a tree instead of a tombstone.

- Members of the Bahá'í Faith are not embalmed. Instead, the body is washed and placed in a cotton, linen or silk shroud. The body is to be buried within one hour's journey from the place of death, if this is feasible. Cremation is also forbidden.

- Traditional Jewish law forbids embalming or cremation, and burial is to be done as soon as possible—preferably within 24 hours. However, under certain circumstances, burial may be delayed if it is impossible to bury a person immediately, or to permit the deceased to be buried in Israel. Guidance of a Rabbi or the local *chevra kadisha* (Jewish Burial Society) should be sought regarding any questions, as particular circumstances may justify leniencies. Notably, the Biblical Joseph was, according to the (Genesis 50:26), embalmed in the Egyptian fashion as was his father Israel (Jacob) (Genesis 50:2). The chevra kadisha ensures the body is guarded (except during the Sabbath); typically these shomrim (guards) recite Psalms within earshot of the deceased. The deceased is dressed in a *kittel*—a white robe-like garment, and then in a white cotton shroud. Burial in Israel is done without a casket. Outside Israel caskets may be used if required by local custom or law, but it must be a simple coffin, made without nails or glue, so as to permit natural processes to process the corpse.

- Embalming is not practiced by Muslims, as they bury their deceased. For them, the body is sacred. They are urged not to delay the burial process. The body is washed usually by a close relative. He or she is then dressed in a clean, perfumed, plain white burial shroud, called "kafan". People gather to hold a joint prayer for the dead called 'Salat Al-Janaza'. They do not use coffins. Instead, the 2 meter deep grave has edging approximately 1 meter down, where a slab is placed which in turn is covered with loose dirt.

• Traditionally Hindus burn the body in proper process.

Notable Embalming

• **Lord Nelson** (1758–1805) was preserved for two months in brandy and spirits of wine mixed with camphor and myrrh after which time the body was found to be in excellent condition and completely plastic.

• **Charles XII**, (1682–1718) is one of several Swedish kings to have been embalmed. When Charles XII's sarcophagus was opened in 1917, his features were still recognizable, almost 200 years after his death. Photographs of his remains clearly show the gunshot wound to his head leading to his death.

• **Pope Saint John XXIII**, body is on display in an altar on the main floor of the Basilica of Saint Peter after having been exhumed from the grottoes beneath the main altar and has retained an extremely well preserved state.

• Murdered civil rights activist **Medgar Evers** was so well embalmed that a viable autopsy was able to be performed on his corpse decades after his death and this helped secure the conviction of his killer.

• Famous Russian surgeon and scientist **NI Pirogov**, was embalmed after his death in 1881. He was embalmed using the technique he himself developed. His body rests in a church in Vinnitsa, Ukraine.

• **Abraham Lincoln** was embalmed after his assassination in 1865. In order to prevent anyone stealing Lincoln's body, Lincoln's eldest son Robert called for Lincoln's exhumation in 1901 to be buried in a concrete vault in the burial room of his tomb in Springfield, Illinois.

• **Diana, Princess of Wales** was embalmed shortly after her death in France in August 1997. The decision to embalm her provoked conspiracy theories that she was pregnant, as the embalming fluid would have destroyed any evidence of fetal presence in her womb. The official explanation for the embalming was that the warm conditions in the chapel of rest where her body was laid out would have speed up the decomposition of the remains.

Embalming and Ethics

The decision of embalming is generally taken by close relatives of the person after his death. In very exceptional cases the person already declares will to use his body for research purpose or dissection purpose in medical institutions after his death. Though there is no clear guidelines regarding embalming and its applications, but due to various movements like body donation scheme by medical institutions, increasing awareness and will of people there is noted positive results. However, in India majority bodies which were used for dissection purpose were obtained as unclaimed bodies collected by police. Nowadays this scenario is changing.

15

Human Rights

LEARNING OBJECTIVES

After reading this chapter student should:
• Be able to define and explain concept of human rights
• Know classification of human rights
• Know about historical aspects of human rights
• Know about International humanitarian law in worldwide scenario
• Know about human rights group in worldwide practices
• Know role of World Health Organization concerned with human rights
• Know about human rights laws and current status in India
• Know about implications of ethical practices and human rights

INTRODUCTION

The fundamental rights which describe the specific standards, principles or norms of human behavior and are regularly protected as legal rights, irrespective of nation, location, religion or any other status are known as **human rights.**

These rights are applicable for everyone irrespective of individual. If these are applicable to all of us, it is our duty to obey their regulations and always act everyday to prevent or damages rights of others.

Nowadays worldwide human rights became one strong movement. NGOs play an important role in establishment of these movements.

HISTORICAL ASPECTS

16th-18th Century

Two major revolutions occurred during the 18th century, in the United States (1776) and in France (1789), leading to the adoption of the United States Declaration of Independence and the French Declaration of the Rights of Man and of the Citizen respectively, both of which established certain legal rights to every human or citizen of country.

Additionally, the Virginia Declaration of Rights of 1776 included into law a number of fundamental civil rights and civil freedoms like freedom of speech, right to live, etc.

19th Century

Over the issue of slavery, in the 19th century it became central point. A number of reformers, notably British Member of Parliament William Wilberforce, worked towards the abolition of the Atlantic slave trade and abolition of slavery.

Many groups and movements have achieved profound social changes over the course of the 20th century in the name of human rights.

The establishment of the International Committee of the Red Cross, the 1864 Lieber Code and the first of the Geneva Conventions in 1864 laid the foundations of International humanitarian law, to be further developed following the two World Wars.

20th Century

The World Wars, and the huge losses of life and gross abuses of human rights that took place during that period, were a driving force behind the development of modern human rights instruments.

At the 1945 Yalta Conference, the Allied Powers agreed to create a new body to supplant the League's role; this was to be the United Nations. The United Nations has played an important role in international human rights law since its creation. Following the World Wars, the United Nations and its members developed much of the discourse and the bodies of law that now make up international humanitarian law and international human rights law.

CLASSIFICATION

At international level human rights has been broadly divided into civil and political rights, and economic, social and cultural rights.

Civil and political rights are described in Articles 3 to 21 of the Universal Declaration of Human Rights (UDHR) and in the International Covenant on Civil and Political Rights (ICCPR). Economic, social and cultural rights are enshrined in Articles 22 to 28 of the Universal Declaration of Human Rights (UDHR) and in the International Covenant on Economic, Social and Cultural Rights (ICESCR).

INDIVISIBILITY

The UDHR included both economic, social and cultural rights and civil and political rights because it was based on the principle that the different rights could only successfully exist in combination.

The ideal of free human beings enjoying civil and political freedom and freedom from fear and want can only be achieved if conditions are created whereby everyone may enjoy his civil and political rights, as well as his social, economic and cultural rights.

— International Covenant on Civil and Political Rights and the International Covenant on Economic, Social and Cultural Rights, 1966

This is held to be true because without civil and political rights the public cannot assert their economic, social and cultural rights. Similarly, without livelihoods and a working society, the public cannot assert or make use of civil or political rights.

The indivisibility and interdependence of all human rights has been confirmed by the 1993 Vienna Declaration and Programme of Action:

All human rights are universal, indivisible and interdependent and related. The international community must treat human rights globally in a fair and equal manner, on the same footing, and with the same emphasis.

— Vienna Declaration and Programme of Action, World Conference on Human Rights, 1993

This statement was again endorsed at the 2005 World Summit in New York (paragraph 121).

INTERNATIONAL HUMANITARIAN LAW

The **Geneva Conventions** came into being between 1864 and 1949 as a result of efforts by Henry Dunant, the founder of the International Committee of the Red Cross. The conventions safeguard the human rights of individuals involved in armed conflict, and build on the Hague Conventions of 1899 and 1907, the international community's first attempt to formalize the laws of war and war crimes in the nascent body of secular international law. The conventions were revised as a result of World War II and readopted by the international community in 1949.

Human Rights Promotion

Human rights continue to be promoted around the world through governmental organizations as well as by nongovernment organizations.

Human Rights Group

International **non-governmental human rights organizations** such as Amnesty International, Human Rights Watch, International Service for Human Rights and FIDH monitor what they see as human rights issues around the world and promote their views on the subject. Human rights organizations have been said to ""translate complex international issues into activities to be undertaken by concerned citizens in their own community". Human rights organizations frequently engage in lobbying and advocacy in an effort to convince the United Nations, supranational bodies and national governments to adopt their policies on human rights. Many human-rights organizations have observer status at the various UN bodies tasked with protecting human rights.

RIGHT TO LIFE

Every human being has the inherent right to life. This right shall be priory protected by law. No one shall be arbitrarily deprived of his life. This is the basic right that every human is eligible for it.

— Article 6.1 of the International Covenant on Civil and Political Rights

The right to life is the essential right that a human being has the right not to be killed by another human being. The concept of a right to life is central to debates on the issues of abortion, capital punishment, euthanasia, self defense and war.

Freedom from Torture

Throughout history, torture has been used as a method of political re-education, interrogation, punishment, and coercion. In addition to state-sponsored torture, individuals or groups may be motivated to inflict torture on others for similar reasons to those of a state; however, the motive for torture can also be for the sadistic gratification of the torturer, as in the Moors murders.

Freedom from Slavery

Freedom from slavery is internationally recognized as a human right. Article 4 of the Universal Declaration of Human Rights states:

No one shall be held in slavery or servitude; slavery and the slave trade shall be prohibited in all their forms.

Despite this, the number of slaves today is higher than at any point in history, remaining as high as 12 million to 27 million. Most are debt slaves, largely in South Asia, who are under debt bondage incurred by lenders, sometimes even for generations.

Human trafficking is primarily for prostitution of women and children into sex industries.

Groups such as the American Anti-Slavery Group, Anti-Slavery International, Free the Slaves, the Anti-Slavery Society, and the Norwegian Anti-Slavery Society continue to campaign to rid the world of slavery.

RIGHT TO A FAIR TRIAL

Everyone is entitled in full equality to a fair and public hearing by an independent and impartial tribunal, in the determination of his rights and obligations and of any criminal charge against him.

The right to a fair trial has been defined in numerous regional and international human rights instruments. It is one of the most extensive human rights and all international human rights instruments enshrine it in more than one article. The right to a fair trial is one of the most litigated human rights and substantial case law has been established on the interpretation of this human right. Despite variations in wording and placement of the various fair trial rights, international human rights instrument define the right to a fair trial in broadly the same terms. The aim of the right is to ensure the proper administration of justice.

Freedom of Speech

Freedom of speech is the freedom to speak freely without censorship. The term freedom of expression is sometimes used synonymously, but includes any act of seeking, receiving and imparting information or ideas, regardless of the medium used.

Freedom of thought, Conscience and Religion

Everyone has the right to freedom of thought, conscience and religion; this right includes freedom to change his religion or belief, and freedom, either alone or in community with others and in public or private, to manifest his religion or belief in teaching, practice, worship and observance.

— Article 18 of the International Covenant on Civil and Political Rights

Freedom of thought, conscience and religion are closely related rights that protect the freedom of an individual or community, in public or private, to think and freely hold conscientious beliefs and to manifest religion or belief in teaching, practice, worship, and observance; the concept is generally recognized also to include the freedom to change religion or not to follow any religion. The freedom to *leave* or discontinue membership in a religion or religious group—in religious terms called "apostasy"—is also a fundamental part of religious freedom, covered by Article 18 of the Universal Declaration of Human Rights.

Freedom of Movement

Freedom of movement asserts that a citizen of a state in which that citizen is present has the liberty to travel, reside in, and/ or work in any part of the state where one pleases within the limits of respect for the liberty and rights of others, and to leave that state and return at any time.

RIGHT TO DEBATE

Events and new possibilities can affect existing rights or require new ones. Advances of technology, medicine, and philosophy constantly challenge the status quo of human rights thinking.

RIGHT TO KEEP AND BEAR ARMS

The right to keep and bear arms for defense is described in the philosophical and political writings of Aristotle, Cicero, John Locke, Machiavelli, the English Whigs and others.

RIGHT TO WATER

The right to water has been recognized in a wide range of international documents, including treaties, declarations and other standards.

SEXUAL AND REPRODUCTIVE RIGHTS

Human rights include women's rights and sexual and reproductive rights. Sexual and reproductive rights are part of a continuum of human rights, which includes the rights to life, health and education, the rights to equality and non-discrimination, and the right to decide the timing, number and spacing of one's children.

The ICPD Program of Action in paragraph 7.2 "defines an individual's sexual and reproductive health as complete well-being related to sexual activity and reproduction. Sexual and reproductive health and rights (SRHR) encompass both entitlements and freedoms. This includes the definition of reproductive rights in paragraph 7.3 of the ICPD PoA, which clarifies that these are not a new set of rights but human rights in existing human rights instruments related to sexual and reproductive autonomy and the attainment of sexual and reproductive health.

WORLD HEALTH ORGANIZATION

Reproductive rights were first established as a subset of human rights at the United Nations 1968 International Conference on Human Rights. The sixteenth article of the resulting Proclamation of Teheran states, "Parents have a basic human right to determine freely and responsibly the number and the spacing of their children."

Reproductive rights may include some or all of the following rights: the right to legal or safe abortion, the right to control one's reproductive functions, the right to quality reproductive healthcare, and the right to education and access in order to make reproductive choices free from coercion, discrimination, and violence.

Reproductive rights may also be understood to include education about contraception and sexually transmitted infections, and freedom from coerced sterilization and contraception, protection from gender-based practices such as female genital cutting (FGC) and male genital mutilation (MGM).

HUMAN RIGHTS IN INDIA

Human rights in India is an issue being complicated by the country's large size, its tremendous diversity, its status as a developing country and as secular, democratic republic. The Constitution of India provides for Fundamental rights, which include freedom of religion. Clauses also provide for freedom of speech, as well as separation of executive and judiciary and freedom of movement within the country and abroad.

In its report on human rights in India during 2013, which was published in 2014, Human Rights Watch stated, "India took positive steps in strengthening laws protecting women and children, and, in several important cases, prosecuting state security forces for extrajudicial killings." The report also condemned the persistent impunity for abuse linked to insurgency in Maoist areas, Jammu and Kashmir, Manipur and

Assam. The report also went on to state, "The fact that the government responded to public outrage confirms India's claims of a vibrant civil society. An independent judiciary and free media also acted as checks on abusive practices. However, reluctance to hold public officials to account for abuses or dereliction of duty continued to foster a culture of corruption and impunity".

On a global level, India opts for a policy of "non-interference in internal affairs of other countries". However, India is engaged in promoting stability and human rights in Afghanistan, pledging nearly US\$2 billion for the country's rehabilitation and reconstruction efforts, supporting education of girls, providing some police training, and granting asylum to a number of activists fleeing Taliban threats.

Until the Delhi High Court decriminalized consensual private sexual acts between consenting adults on 2 July 2009, homosexuality was considered criminal as per interpretations of the ambiguous Section 377 of the 150-year-old Indian Penal Code (IPC), a law passed by the colonial British authorities. However, this law was very rarely enforced. In its ruling decriminalizing homosexuality, the Delhi High Court noted that existed law conflicted with the fundamental rights guaranteed by the Constitution of India, and such criminalising is violative of Articles 21, 14 and 15 of the Constitution.

On 11 December 2013, homosexuality was again criminalized by a Supreme Court ruling.

Around 10,000 Nepali women are brought to India annually for commercial sexual exploitation. Each year 20,000–25,000 women and children are trafficked from Bangladesh.

Along with international human trafficking there is also statewide illegal human trafficking in India mainly for the purpose of commercial sexual exploitation. Mumbai and Kolkata are major hubs for such purpose.

Religious violence is another tragedy finds in India.

16

Immortality

LEARNING OBJECTIVES

After reading this chapter student should:

- Be able to define and explain concept of immortality
- Be able to explain concept of cryonics, cybernetics and virtual life
- Understand concept of biological immortality
- Understand different religious views concerned with immortality
- Know about current experiments in immortality
- Understand values of ethics and immortality

INTRODUCTION

Immortality is eternal life or the ability to live forever.

Any living element has natural limitation of life span. No science has power to overcome it. Numbers of scientists are currently working over this fact; however, some success is advocated for life extension rather than immortality.

Aubrey de Grey, a scientist has developed proposed programme known as **SENS**, a series of biomedical rejuvenation strategies to reverse human aging, which can be implementable in future.

In the future, with sufficient medical advancements and life extension technologies dead can be revived which is a dream of human.

RELIGION AND IMMORTALITY

Life after death is the basic fundamental concept explained in various religious literatures including Hinduism, Buddhism, Christians, Islam, etc. However, the concept of soul is used differently by different religions.

ALCHEMY

Alchemy is simply nothing but physical immortality where person can maintain cautious thought with existence in physical form. It can be based on various scientific methods like cryonics, rejuvenation, etc.

DEATH AND FACTS

There are basically three major reasons behind death—**ageing, disease and trauma.**

Aubrey de Grey, defines aging as "a collection of cumulative changes to the molecular and cellular structure of an adult organism, which result in essential metabolic processes, but which also, once they progress far enough, increasingly disrupt metabolism, resulting in pathology and death."

Major cause of death may be unreserved cell loss.

Disease is an abnormal condition affecting body of an organism.

Trauma is third major cause of death either due to any evidence or any situation that damages living organism.

Biological Immortality

Biological immortality is a condition where cell or organism does not experience ageing or death.

As the existence of biologically immortal species demonstrates, there is no thermodynamic necessity for senescence: a defining feature of life is that it takes in free energy from the environment and unloads its entropy as waste.

Modern theories on the evolution of aging include the following:

• **Mutation accumulation (1952)** is a theory postulated by **Peter Medawar** to explain how evolution would select for aging. Essentially, aging is never selected against, as organisms have offspring before the mortal mutations surface in an individual.

- **Antagonistic pleiotropy** (1957) is a theory proposed as an alternative by George C. Williams, a critic of Medawar . In antagonistic pleiotropy, genes carry effects that are both beneficial and detrimental. In essence this refers to genes that offer benefits early in life, but exact a cost later on, i.e. decline and death.

- **The disposable soma theory** was proposed (1977) by Thomas Kirkwood, which states that an individual body must allocate energy for metabolism, reproduction, and maintenance, and must compromise when there is food scarcity. Compromise in allocating energy to the repair function is what causes the body gradually to deteriorate with age, according to Kirkwood.

CRYONICS

Cryonics is the process by which storming the organisms at cryogenic temperatures where complete stoppage of metabolism and decaying process, which is used for preserving organisms.

VIRTUAL LIFE

By using computer memory and program system, the person's personality and memory are feeds to computer along with human consciousness, so that future virtual interaction with same human is possible.

Another possible mechanism for mind upload is to obtain a detailed scan of an individual's original, organic brain and simulate the entire structure in a computer.

CYBERNETICS

Transforming a human into a cyborg can include brain implants or extracting a human mind and placing it in a robotic life-support system. Even replacing biological organs with robotic ones could increase life span (i.e. pacemakers) and depending on the definition, many technological upgrades to the body, like genetic modifications or the addition of nanobots would qualify an individual as a cyborg. Such modifications would make one impervious to aging and disease and theoretically immortal unless killed or destroyed.

EVOLUTIONARY IMMORTALITY

As the natural tendency is to create progressively more complex structures, there will be a time, when evolution of a more complex human brain will be faster via a process of developmental singularity rather than through Darwinian evolution.

ANCIENT GREEK RELIGION

Immortality in ancient Greek religion originally always included an eternal union of body and soul as can be seen in Homer, Hesiod, and various other ancient texts. The soul was considered to have an eternal existence in Hades, but without the body the soul was considered dead.

Buddhism

The goal of Hinayana is Arhatship and Nirvana. By contrast, the goal of Mahayana is Buddhahood.

According to one Tibetan Buddhist teaching, Dzogchen, individuals can transform the physical body into an immortal body of light called the rainbow body.

Christianity

Christian theology holds that Adam and Eve lost physical immortality for themselves and all their descendants in the Fall of Man, although this initial "imperishability of the bodily frame of man" was "a preternatural condition". Christians who profess the Nicene Creed believe that every dead person (whether they believed in Christ or not) will be resurrected from the dead at the Second Coming, and this belief is known as Universal resurrection.

NT Wright, a theologian and former Bishop of Durham, has said many people forget the physical aspect of what Jesus promised. He told Time: "Jesus' resurrection marks the beginning of a restoration that he will complete upon his return.

Part of this will be the resurrection of all the dead, who will 'awake', be embodied and participate in the renewal. Wright says John Polkinghorne, a physicist and a priest, has put it this way: 'God will download our software onto his hardware until the time he gives us new hardware to run the software again for ourselves.' That gets to two things nicely: that the period after death (the Intermediate state) is a period when we are in God's presence but not active in our own bodies, and also that the more important transformation will be when we are again embodied and administering Christ's kingdom."

Hinduism

Hindus believe in an immortal soul which is reincarnated after death. According to Hinduism, people repeat a process of life, death, and rebirth in a cycle called samsara. If they live their life well, their *karma* improves and their station in the next life will be higher, and conversely lower if they live their life poorly. After many life times of perfecting its karma, the soul is freed from the cycle and lives in perpetual bliss. There is no place of eternal torment in Hinduism, although if a soul consistently lives very evil lives, it could work its way down to the very bottom of the cycle.

There are explicit renderings in the Upanishads alluding to a physically immortal state brought about by purification, and sublimation of the 5 elements that make up the body. For example, in the Shvetashvatara Upanishad (Chapter 2, Verse 12), it is stated "When earth, water fire, air and akasa arise, that is to say, when the five attributes of the elements, mentioned in the books on yoga, become manifest then the yogi's body becomes purified by the fire of yoga and he is free from illness, old age and death." This phenomenon is possible when the soul reaches enlightenment while the body and mind are still intact, an extreme rarity, and can only be achieved upon the highest most dedication, meditation and consciousness.

To Maharishi Mahesh Yogi, the verse means, "Once a man has become established in the understanding of the permanent reality of life, his mind rises above the influence of pleasure and pain. Such an unshakable man passes beyond the influence of death and in the permanent phase of life: he attains eternal life ... A man established in the understanding of the unlimited abundance of absolute existence is naturally free from existence of the relative order. This is what gives him the status of immortal life."

Judaism

The traditional concept of an immaterial and immortal soul distinct from the body was not found in Judaism before the Babylonian Exile, but developed as a result of interaction with Persian and Hellenistic philosophies. The only Hebrew word traditionally translated "soul" (*nephesh*) in English language Bibles refers to a living, breathing conscious body, rather than to an immortal soul. In the New Testament, the Greek word traditionally translated "soul" has substantially the same meaning as the Hebrew, without reference to an immortal soul. 'Soul' may refer to the whole person.

Taoism

In the Tractate of Actions and their Retributions, a traditional teaching, spiritual immortality can be rewarded to people who do a certain amount of good deeds and live a simple, pure life. A list of good deeds and sins are tallied to determine whether or not a mortal is worthy. Spiritual immortality in this definition allows the soul to leave the earthly realms of afterlife and go to pure realms in the Taoist cosmology.

Ethics of Immortality

The possibility of clinical immortality raises a host of medical, philosophical, and religious issues and ethical questions. These include persistent vegetative states, the nature of personality over time, technology to mimic or copy the mind or its processes, social and economic disparities created by longevity, and survival of the heat death of the universe.

The Epic of Gilgamesh, one of the first literary works, is primarily a quest of a hero seeking to become immortal.

UNDESIRABILITY OF IMMORTALITY

Physical immortality has also been imagined as a form of eternal torment, as in Mary Shelley's short story **"The Mortal Immortal"**, the protagonist of which witnesses everyone he cares about dying around him. Jorge Luis Borges explored the idea that life gets its meaning from death in the short story "The Immortal"; an entire society having achieved immortality, they found time becoming infinite, and so found no motivation for any action. In his book "Thursday's Fictions", and the stage and film adaptations of it, Richard James Allen tells the story of a woman named Thursday who tries to cheat the cycle of reincarnation to get a form of eternal life. At the end of this fantastical tale, her son, Wednesday, who has witnessed the havoc his mother's quest has caused, forgoes the opportunity for immortality when it is offered to him. Likewise, the novel Tuck Everlasting depicts immortality as "falling off the wheel of life" and is viewed as a curse as opposed to a blessing.

IMMORTALITY AND ETHICS

The increasing practices and research concern towards immortality and dream of human to be live forever are two issues going together for the sake of their target. Anti-aging concern modern medicine research and its implantation in near future and simultaneously maintain our morals will be our prime focus. Patient autonomy and his rights should be our priority. Though there will be availability of advance drugs that can increases our cell lives thousands times but can we think issues arises due to such life on earth. It is question of debate that immortality will be curse or blessing by modern medicine to human.

Medical Futility

LEARNING OBJECTIVES

After reading this chapter student should:
• Be able to define and explain concept of medical futility
• Know about classification of medical futility
• Understand values of ethics in medical futility
• Know about controversial facts concerned with medical futility

INTRODUCTION

Medical futility has been an important topic in medical bioethics. Medical futility is based on the fact that if there is no chance of patient survival, then why advanced treatment should be provided to the patient? Some of these cases are examined in courts of various countries.

Patient wish or consent is prime important factor in this context. When patient is unable to opt for consent, his relatives can be asked for such provisions. In some hospitals, medical futility is referred to as "non-beneficial care."

Baby Doe Law establishes state protection for a disabled child's right to life, ensuring that this right is protected even over the wishes of parents or guardians in cases where they want to withhold treatment.

Both legal and moral values are important during such situations or decision making states by clinician.

Medical futility may be broadly classified into two parts, viz. **Quantitative futility** and **qualitative futility.** Quantitative futility stands for where the stated intervention benefit the patient is exceedingly poor, while qualitative futility stands for where the quality of benefit an intervention will produce is exceedingly poor.

Here we want to know clearly futility is not a issue concern with medical treatment but is associated with particular intervention at a particular time, for a specific patient.

MEDICAL FUTILITY AND ETHICAL APPROACH

It is patient right to chose treatment which he wish. Our duty is to cure the patient or take him away from pain. The clinician should think which treatment protocol will be better for his patient. Such treatments that cause pain or leads to poor quality life in last days of patient, discomfort in final days, false hope of his relatives should rethink by the clinician.

Generally the term medical futility applies when, based on medical data and professional experience, a treating healthcare provider determines that an intervention is no longer beneficial. While physicians have the ethical authority to withhold or withdraw medically futile interventions, communicating with professional colleagues involved in a patient's care, and with patients and family, greatly improves the experience and outcome for all.

What if the patient or family requests an intervention that the healthcare team considers futile?

You have a duty as a physician to communicate openly with the patient or family members about interventions that are being withheld or withdrawn and to explain the rationale for such decisions. The aim of respectful communication should be to elicit the patient's goals, explain the goals of treatment, and help patients and families understand how particular medical interventions would help or hinder their goals and the goals of treatment. It is important to approach such conversations with compassion.

In some instances, it may be appropriate to continue temporarily to make a futile intervention available in order to assist the patient or family in coming to terms with the gravity of their situation and reaching closure. For example, a futile intervention for a terminally ill patient may in some instances be continued temporarily in order to allow time for a loved one arriving from another state to see the patient for the last time. However, futile interventions should not be used for the benefit of family members if this is likely to cause the patient substantial suffering, or if the family's interests are clearly at odds with those of the patient.

If intractable conflict arises, a fair process for conflict resolution should occur. Involvement of an ethics consultation service is desirable in such situations. The 1999 Texas Advance Directives Act provides one model for designing a fair process for conflict resolution.

MEDICAL FUTILITY AND RATIONING

Futility refers to the benefit of a particular intervention for a particular patient. With futility, the central question is not, "How much money does this treatment cost?" or, "Who else might benefit from it?" but instead, "Does the intervention have any reasonable prospect of helping this patient?"

MEDICAL FUTILITY AND PATIENT AGE

Futility has no necessary correlation with a patient's age. What determines whether a treatment is futile, whether or not the treatment benefits the patient. In cases where evidence clearly shows that older patients have poorer outcomes than younger patients, age may be a reliable indicator of patient benefit, but it is benefit, not age, that supports a judgment of medical futility. For patients of all ages, healthcare professionals should advocate for medically beneficial care, and refrain from treatments that do not help the patient.

MEDICAL FUTILITY AND CONTROVERSY

While medical futility is a well-established basis for withdrawing and withholding treatment, it has also been the source of ongoing debate. One source of controversy centers on the exact definition of medical futility, which continues to be debated in the scholarly literature. Second, an appeal to medical futility is sometimes understood as giving unilateral decision-making authority to physicians at the bedside. Proponents of medical futility reject this interpretation, and argue that properly understood futility should reflect a professional consensus, which ultimately accepted by the wider society that physicians serve. Third, in the clinical setting, an appeal to "futility" can sometimes function as a conversation stopper. Thus, some clinicians find that even when the concept applies, the language of "futility" is best avoided in discussions with patients and families. Likewise, some professionals have dispensed with the term "medical futility" and replaced it with other language, such as "medically inappropriate." Finally, an appeal to medical futility can create the false impression that medical decisions are value-neutral and based solely on the physician's scientific expertise. Yet clearly this is not the case. The physician's goal of helping the sick is itself a value stance and all medical decision making incorporates values.

18

Oncofertility

LEARNING OBJECTIVES

After reading this chapter student should:
• Be able to define and explain concept of oncofertility
• Know about scope of oncofertility in men, women and in pediatrics
• Understands financial, legal and ethical considerations in oncofertility
• Know about status of oncofertility in India and limitations

INTRODUCTION

Oncofertility is the term especially designed the options which expand possibilities of reproduction in cancer survivor patients.

The term coined by **Dr Teresa K. Woodruff** at the Oncofertility Consortium in 2006.

During cancer treatment either by chemotherapy, radiotherapy or surgery option, most of the time these may destroy patient's ability to have children in later life. Oncofertility research focuses towards such issues that may increasing fertility preservation options.

This is nowadays major societal issue in clinical practice.

Oncofertility incorporates reproductive issues after cancer treatment, such as family planning, complex contraception, hormonal management throughout survivorship, surrogacy, and adoption, etc.

FERTILITY OPTIONS FOR MEN

Established fertility preservation options for men include Sperm Banking in which a semen sample is produced, frozen, and stored for future use and testicular sperm extraction during which sperm is retrieved directly from the testes through a short surgery and frozen. Experimental options include Testicular Tissue Banking when testicular tissue is surgically removed and frozen. Scientists are developing methods to use this tissue for fertility preservation in males.

Men who do not preserve their feritlity prior to cancer treatment may have children through Donor Sperm using sperm from a known or anonymous donor to achieve a pregnancy with a female partner using assisted reproductive technologies or adoption by permanently assuming all rights and responsibilities of a child through a legal process.

FERTILITY OPTIONS FOR WOMEN

Options for women to have children after cancer have increased significantly in recent years.

Women should be counseled on established options such as embryo banking in which hormonal stimulation causes the production of multiple eggs, which are removed, fertilized by sperm, and frozen for future use, and egg banking in which hormonal stimulation causes the production of multiple eggs, which are removed and frozen for storage and future use, and Ovarian Transposition and Shielding in which ovaries can be surgically moved or shielded from the area receiving radiation.

This technique does not protect against the effects of chemotherapy.

Experimental techniques include ovarian tissue banking in which an ovary is surgically removed and frozen to be transplanted back into the woman when she is ready to have children.

Scientists are also working on ways to mature undeveloped eggs from this ovarian tissue. After sterilizing cancer treatment, a woman can also choose surrogacy when a woman carries a pregnancy for another woman or couple or adoption. Recent efforts also investigate the implications of a cancer diagnosis during pregnancy.

FERTILITY OPTIONS FOR CHILDREN

Prepubescent children have fewer options to preserve fertility than adults. These include testicular sperm extraction for males and ovarian tissue banking for females.

FINANCIAL, ETHICAL, AND LEGAL CONSIDERATIONS

Fertility preservation costs may be prohibitive for young patients and multiple organizations now provide methods to reduce costs for patients. These include Fertile Hope and Fertile Action.

In 2011, California State Assembly Bill 428 was introduced to mandate insurance companies to provide healthcare coverage for fertility preservation. In addition, the Supreme Court of the United States addressed the Social Security implications of oncofertility in March, 2012 with Astrue vs. Capato.

Research also investigates ethical issues in oncofertility, such as the decision-making process for adolescent children and their families.

INDIA AND ONCOFERTILITY

In India, oncofertility research is in embryonic stage. However, alternative practices such as hormonal management throughout survivorship, surrogacy, and adoption are routinely used. In some center, formation of sperm banks, test tube baby concept is in reality.

Though afterwards there is vast scope to this concept. There is need of motivation and funding from government or nongovernment sector. Ethical counseling is one of the important issues in this matter.

19

Dichotomy and Prudence

LEARNING OBJECTIVES

After reading this chapter student should:

- Be able to define and explain concept of dichotomy and prudence
- Know about scope and implications of dichotomy and prudence
- Know about prudence and malpractice in India and ethical approaches

INTRODUCTION

Dichotomy and prudence are two important concepts in medical ethics.

These are mainly concerned with grounds to choice of tests and right to refusal of tests by the patient. It is an acceptable fact that patient has choice for test selection as well as right to refuse that test under his autonomy. But in emergency the same situation may be demined and clinician decides best for patient under basic traditional principles of medical bioethics. That time dichotomy and prudence are two important virtues play vital role.

In conclusion if right to choice of test is patient autonomy, simultaneously best test selection from clinician under beneficence is doctor's duty which are both, viz. autonomy and beneficence, basic traditional principles of medical bioethics.

DICHOTOMY

In general sense, dichotomy is the process or practice of making two contradictory groups.

In clinical context the word dichotomy can synonymously be used for difference in opinion of doctor. Very simply, in emergency, the decision of admission of patient or referral to other higher specialty for his benefit has to be solved by doctor.

Dichotomy can simply be classified into true dichotomy and false dichotomy.

True dichotomy is condition, where a decision is based on a fact that there may be some middle way other than these two options only.

False dichotomy is a condition, where a decision is based on a fact or belief and at that time forgetting that there may be some other ways.

In clinical practice these principles or judgments are very important.

Especially in emergency room, when doctors decides that this is an emergency, the decision of choice of therapy or drugs is solely in hands of doctors either due to time being factor.

The matching with ethical issues, patient autonomy, permission from his relatives or opting such necessary permission from ethical committee is secondary at that time.

PRUDENCE (LATIN: PRUDENTIA)

Prudence is classically considered to be a virtue, is the ability to govern and discipline oneself by the use of reason.

It can be used synonymous with cautiousness.

Actually this word derives from the 14th-century old French word prudence, which, in turn, derives from the Latin **prudentia** meaning "foresight, sagacity".

It is often associated with wisdom, insight, and knowledge.

While considering values of prudence in clinical practice, the ability to judge between virtuous and vicious actions, not only in a common sense, but with concern to appropriate actions at a given time and place is very important.

The choice of tests as diagnostic value, decided by clinician when patient admitted to him. The values of these tests, their usefulness in diagnosis, patient affordability, alternative tests, time, easy availability of tests, needfulness, etc. are very important issues.

A basic principle of bioethics plays an important role in this regard. While offering to these tests, the doctor should respect the autonomy of the patient. Beneficence is another issue, which is base of bioethics. The doctor should choose the tests that judgments will provide justice with patient.

Hence prudence of choice of tests and refusal to test by patient is very practical issue in clinical practice.

Sole knowledge of doctor and his ethical approach play a vital role in this context.

PRUDENCE AND MALPRACTICE IN INDIA

Nowadays due to decrease in ethical values and rat race competition choice of tests are not from patient point of view but from doctor's beneficence has increased. A simple example, when patient admitted to any hospital, that hospital makes compulsion for tests, from where these should be carried out, from whom these should be done, etc. This leads to one of major open sources for cut practice and fees splitting issues.

Medical Council of India and other regulatory authorities made strict clauses against such issue.

Ethical education in medical curriculum is the step opted by MCI in this regard.

20

Animal Ethics

"The greatness of a nation can be judged by the way its animals are treated."

— Mahatma Gandhi

LEARNING OBJECTIVES

After reading this chapter student should:
• Be able to define and explain concept of animal ethics
• Know about scope of animal ethics
• Know about different movements of animal ethics in India
• Know about animal rights and animal laws in India
• Know about guidelines for use of Laboratory animals in Medical Colleges under CPCSEA Laws

INTRODUCTION

Animal ethics is a term used to describe human–animal relationships and how animals ought to be treated during research activity.

Animal ethics includes area of ethical animal handling, animals living condition standards, animal rights and animal law. Ethical handling of animals means to respect them as individual. All basic principles of medical bioethics are applicable to animals. In ethical handling practices there are a number of regulations implemented by various countries as per their need. But the common issue in all of them is to prevent pain or injury to animals.

ANIMAL RIGHTS AND ANIMAL LAWS IN INDIA

The Prevention of Cruelty to Animals Act, 1960 is an Act of the Parliament of India enacted to prevent the infliction of unnecessary pain or suffering of animals and to amend the laws relating to the prevention of cruelty to animals. As per the provisions of the law the Government of India formed the Animal Welfare Board of India.

The **Animal Welfare Board of India** is a statutory advisory body advising the Government of India on animal welfare laws, and promotes animal welfare in the country of India. It works to ensure that animal welfare laws in the country are followed; provides grants to Animal Welfare Organizations; and considers itself "the face of the animal welfare movement in the country".

Concerned about the abuse of animals in research, in the Board's early history, it recommended that the government create the Committee for the Purpose of Control and Supervision of Experiments on Animals (CPCSEA). The Committee was created, and the Board's representative Dr S Chinny Krishna deposed twice before the Committee about "the dismal state of laboratories in India".

PETA India, which based in Mumbai, was launched in January 2000. PETA India operates under the simple principle that animals are not ours to eat, wear, experiment on or use for entertainment, while educating policymakers and the public about animal abuse and promoting an understanding of the right of all animals to be treated with respect.

PETA India focusses primarily on the areas in which the greatest numbers of animals suffer the most: in the food and leather industries, in laboratories and in the entertainment industry. PETA India's investigative work, public education efforts, research, animal rescues, legislative work, special events, celebrity involvement and national media coverage have resulted in countless improvements to the quality of life for animals and have saved countless animals' lives.

Maneka Gandhi is a famous environmentalist and animal rights leader in India. She has earned international awards and acclaim for her contribution and constant work in issue concerned with animal rights. She was appointed chairwoman of the Committee for the Purpose of Control and Supervision of Experiments on Animals (CPCSEA) in 1995. Under her direction, CPCSEA members carried unannounced inspections of laboratories where animals are used for scientific research.

She has filed Public Interest Litigations that have achieved the replacement of the municipal killing of homeless dogs with a sterilisation programme, the unregulated sale of airguns and a ban on mobile or travelling zoos. She currently chairs the Jury of International Energy Globe Foundation which meets annually in Austria to award the best environmental innovations of the year. She is a member of the Eurosolar Board and the Wuppertal Institute, Germany.

She started the gathering people for Animals rights in 1992 and it is the largest organisation for animal rights/welfare in India. Maneka Gandhi is also a patron of International Animal Rescue. She is a vegan and has advocated this lifestyle on ethical and health grounds. She also anchored a weekly television program named "Heads and Tails" highlighting sufferings meted out to animals due to their commercial exploitation. She has also authored a book under the same title. Her other books were about Indian people names. She is a cast member for the documentary "A Delicate Balance".

World animal day, as 4 October was started in 1931 at a convention of ecologists in Florence.

Guidelines for use of Laboratory animals in Medical Colleges under "Purpose of Control and Supervision of Experiments on Animals" (CPCSEA) Laws

Guidelines for use of Laboratory animals in Medical Colleges preface laboratory animals used in medical colleges play an important role in teaching/research as well as developing skills for diagnosis.

Here the animal is almost exclusively used as a substitute or model for man as most laboratory animals have the same set of organs heart, lungs, liver and so on which work in the same way as they do in humans. Knowledge gained from animal experiments enhances the understanding of the subjects like physiology, microbiology, pharmacology, biochemistry, etc.

Animal experiments give an insight to the students about the etiology, diagnosis, progression and methods of prevention of various diseases.

Commonly used animals in medical colleges are frogs, rats, mice, rabbits, guinea pigs, cats, dogs, monkeys and to a lesser extent sheep. Use of defined animals in appropriate conditions will reduce the stress on the animals and will result in generating reproducible and reliable results. A thorough knowledge of the biological characteristics and husbandry requirements of the species to be used is essential to ensure animal welfare. It is obligatory on the part of investigators/students to handle the animals gently, following the guidelines of ethical consideration for animal use. These guidelines provide the basic minimum provisions for animal care in medical colleges using animals for teaching/research purposes and those where breeding of such animals is also undertaken. It is hoped that the medical fraternity will find these guidelines useful to ensure the welfare of the animals.

PROCUREMENT OF ANIMALS

It will be economical to procure animals from reliable sources rather than breeding them if the requirement of animals is minimal.

The various species of animals required for medical colleges should be procured from recognized sources.

Local procurement sources should be identified by the medical colleges for the supply of non-laboratory bred animals. Medical Colleges with breeding facilities, should procure the breeding stock from a reliable source for initiating a colony ensuring that genetic makeup and health status of animals is known.

Additionally the following aspects has to be taken care of:

1. Healthy animals should be obtained from a recognized source.

2. Acceptable methods and norms of transportation should be followed, considering the distance, seasonal and climatic conditions and the species of animals.

3. The animals should be given a reasonable period for physiological, psychological and nutritional stabilization before their use.

ANIMALS FEEDING

Animals should be fed palatable, non-contaminated, and nutritionally adequate food. Feed should be procured from reliable source. Good quality feed and water should be provided. Areas in which feed are processed or stored should be kept clean and enclosed to prevent entry of insects and wild rodents. Watering devices, such as drinking tubes, should be examined routinely to ensure their proper operation. Feeders should allow easy access to food and watery while minimising contaminating by urine and feces.

SANITATION AND CLEANLINESS

Animal rooms, corridors, storage spaces, and other areas should be cleaned with appropriate detergents and disinfectants. Animals should be kept dry except for those species whose natural habitation need water. Where larger animals and non-human primates are housed soiled litter material should be removed routinely.

Cages should be cleaned each time before animals are placed in them. Animal cages, racks and accessory equipment, such as feeders and watering devices, should be washed and cleaned frequently to keep them free from contamination. ¾ Cages, water bottles, sipper tubes, stoppers and other watering equipment should be washed and disinfected regularly.

Deodorisers or chemical agents other than germicides should not be used to mask animal odors.

VETERINARY CARE

Wherever required, adequate veterinary care must be provided under the supervision and guidance of a registered veterinarian or a person trained and experienced in laboratory animal sciences. Animals should be observed regularly and problems of animal health and behavior, recorded and addressed.

For animals kept for experiments of longer duration, the following steps should be adopted: All animals should be observed for signs of illness, injury or abnormal behavior by the animal house staff and reported to the attending veterinarian. ¾ Diseased animals should be isolated from healthy ones.

Personnel Hygiene and Staff Training

Initial in-house training should be imparted to the staff associated with animals facility. Appropriate and protective gears (gloves, masks, head cover, coat, shoes, etc.) be used by the personnel in the animal facility as per requirement. Personnel should have periodic medical check ups to ensure their health status.

Surgical procedures and duration of experiment: Multiple surgical procedures on an animal for any experiment are not to be practiced unless specified in a protocol.

Restraint

Devices, wherever required, suitable in size and design for holding animals for examination and collection of samples should be made available to minimize stress and avoid injury to the animals and handlers.

RECORDS KEEPING

1. Animal House plan—Name and addresses of the staff including the facility incharge and contact telephone nos.
2. Health records of staff—Training record of staff involved in animal care and procedures.
3. Records pertaining to the items in stock.
4. Animal stock procurement and supply register.
5. Records of experiments or procedures conducted with the number of animals used in each experiment.
6. Clinical record of sick animals and any treatment administered.
7. Mortality and ailing record.

ANESTHESIA AND EUTHANASIA

The scientists should ensure that the procedures which are considered painful are conducted under appropriate anesthesia as recommended for each species of animals. It must also be ensured that the anesthesia is administered to sustain for the full duration of experiment and at no stage the animal is conscious to perceive pain during the experiment.

Animals during post recovery period should be housed individually till they recover fully from the surgical stress.

Euthanasia: The procedure should be carried out quickly and painlessly in an atmosphere free from fear or anxiety. The choice of a method will depend on the nature of study, the species of animal and number of animals to be sacrificed.

The method should in all cases meet the following requirements.

Death: Without causing anxiety, pain or distress with minimum time lag phase.

Minimum physiological and psychological disturbances.

Compatibility with the purpose of study and minimum emotional effect on the operator.

Location should be separated from animal rooms, method should be reliable, safe to the personnel and simple and economical.

Animal House

Animal houses should be made of durable and preferably moisture-proof material and should have adequate space to facilitate free movement of personnel as well as equipment.

Doors should be rust and vermin roof with provision for door closure. Rodent barriers should be provided at all entry points of animal houses.

Walls and ceilings should be free of cracks.

Floors should be smooth, non-absorbent and skid proof.

Temperature and humidity in animal facilities should be controlled for the comfort of the laboratory animals. As far as possible the usage of smaller animal during the extreme weather conditions should be avoided.

Proper lighting system with adequate illumination at cage level should be maintained in the animal room.

The animal cages should provide adequate space to permit freedom of movement and normal postural adjustments, and have a resting place appropriate to the species; provide a comfortable environment; have an escape-proof enclosure that confines animal safely; have easy access to food and water; provide adequate ventilation; meet the biological needs of the animals; keep the animals dry and clean, be consistent with species requirements. However, aquatic animals like frogs and toads need to be kept in clean water free from chlorine and copper, preferably in containers attached to running tap water to prevent the accumulation of waste products.

Houses, pens, boxes, shelves, perches, and other furnishings should be constructed in a manner and made of materials that allow cleaning or replacement in accordance with generally accepted husbandry practices.

Physical separation of animals by species, wherever possible, is recommended to prevent inter-species disease transmission and to eliminate anxiety and possible physiolgoical and behavioral changes due to inter-species conflict.

Population density and group composition should be maintained as stable as possible, particularly for canines, non-human primates, and other social mammals.

Animal facilities should be maintained free from pests and vermins bedding.

Bedding wherever prescribed, should be absorbent, free of toxic chemicals or other substances that could injure animals or personnel.

Bedding should be removed and replaced with fresh materials as often as necessary to keep the animals clean and dry.

21

Medical Research Ethics

LEARNING OBJECTIVES

After reading this chapter student should:

- Be able to define and explain concept of medical research ethics
- Know about scope and current practices of medical research ethics
- Know about structure of ethical committees in India
- Know about values of ethics in research publications
- Know concept of "conflict of interest"
- Understand importance of internet/online sources in research publications

INTRODUCTION

Medical research ethics is one of central areas of interest in current scenario. Nowadays it is conflict that either autonomy first or beneficence first, both which are important principles of ethics. However, these conflicts can be solved or traceable with proper communication. The increasing market of research played a vital role behind this controversy of ethical principles.

In medical research, the Nuremberg Code set a base international standard in 1947, which continued to develop, for example, in response to the ethical violation in the Holocaust. Nowadays, medical research is overseen by an ethics committee that also oversees the informed consent process.

As the medical guidelines established in the Nuremberg Code were imported into the ethical guidelines for the social sciences, informed consent became a common part of the research procedure.

However, while informed consent is the default in medical settings, it is not always required in the social science.

Here, research often involves low or no risk for participants, unlike in many medical experiments. Second, the mere knowledge that they participate in a study can cause people to alter their behavior, as in the Hawthorne Effect: "In the typical lab experiment, subjects enter an environment in which they are keenly aware that their behavior is being monitored, recorded, and subsequently scrutinized."

In such cases, seeking informed consent directly interferes with the ability to conduct the research, because the very act of revealing that a study is being conducted is likely to alter the behavior studied. List exemplifies the potential dilemma that can result: "if one were interested in exploring whether, and to what extent, race or gender influences the prices that buyers pay for used cars, it would be difficult to measure accurately the degree of discrimination among used car dealers who know that they are taking part in an experiment." In cases where such interference is likely, and after careful consideration, a researcher may forgo the informed consent process. This is commonly done after weighting the risk to study participants versus the benefit to society and whether participants are present in the study out of their own wish and treated fairly. Researchers often consult with an Ethics Committee or institutional review board to render a decision.

The birth of new online media, such as social media, has complicated the idea of informed consent.

In an online environment people pay a little attention to Terms of Use agreements and can subject themselves to research without thorough knowledge. This issue came to the public light following a study conducted by Facebook in 2014 and published by Facebook and Cornell University. Facebook conducted a study where they altered the Facebook News Feeds of roughly 700,000 users to reduce either the amount of positive or negative posts they saw for a week. The study then analyzed if the users status updates changed during the different conditions. The study was published in the Proceedings of the National Academy of Sciences.

The lack of informed consent led to outrage among many researchers and users.

The Facebook study controversy raises numerous questions about informed consent and the differences in the ethical review process between publicly- and privately-funded research. Some say Facebook was within its limits and others see the need for more informed consent and/or the establishment of in-house private review boards.

RESEARCH ETHICS

Research ethics is an important area especially concern with scientific research work. It involves a number of fundamentals and principles.

Scientific misconduct such as fraud, data fabrication and plagiarism, etc. are newer issues.

Whistelblowing, education of ethical practices and strict regulatory laws can minimize frequency of such misconducts.

IMPORTANCE OF COMMUNICATION

Communication breakdowns between patients and doctors, between family members, or between members of the medical community, can all lead to disagreements and strong feelings. These breakdowns should be remedied, and many apparently insurmountable "ethics" problems can be solved with open lines of proper communication. This proper communication and well reputed accreditation of hospitals which ensures benchmark bioethics practices should be one important criterion behind it.

There are a number of guidelines which clarify or define clearly the scope of ethics in clinical practice. Declaration of Helsinki is an important guideline delivers authority in human research ethics.

Ethics Committees

For proper communication and regulation there is a need of well-structured committee. These committees are formed by experts including social workers, philosophers, lay people, etc. The number of members, involvement from various fields, their qualifications, etc. are decided by either government or governing bodies, universities, etc.

Nowadays institutional ethics committee approvals are mandatory for publication of any form of research work carried by professionals in reputed or indexed journals. When authors submit their research work proposal for publication, it is accepted that author has gone through process of approval of his topic from institutional ethics committee from his university or institute.

In India, this is mandatory, however it is malpractice that many research workers does not convey their work to institutional ethics committee and publish their work in average quality journals.

MEDICAL ETHICS AND INTERNET

In view of exposure towards internet, researchers from healthcare sector are using internet data for their writing. Majority of International Journals are online available as free of costs in full text format. There are a number of database dedicated for these free services for the benefits of authors like Open J Gate, Jenamics, Aristimax Turkey, etc. It is our moral responsibility to cite that specified work. Whenever researchers use these references, it is mandatory to provide sufficient citations for their work. Otherwise, these works will be considered as plagiarized.

Plagiarism is a major issue born due to lack of knowledge of proper citations. There are a number of free software available over internet to check plagiarism content of your research work. Viper is the best and trusted online software for checking your content before sending to any publication. The process of checking is very easy and self explaining. However, there is a lack of awareness about such checking process, validation from institutions, etc.

In developed countries it is routine practice to plagiarism check for every article submitted for initial proposal. There are notified punishments for such mistakes from their universities.

Along with plagiarism, conflict of interest (disclosure of information) is another important issue.

• Informed consent and privacy are two important ethical values that have to be kept in mind.

• Source of support is also an important addition. It is mandatory to disclose any financial help or support for that work which may or may not have influence over results, etc.

Cultural Concerns

Culture differences can create difficult medical ethics problems. Some cultures have spiritual or magical theories about the origins of disease, for example, and reconciling these beliefs with the tenets of Western medicine can be difficult.

Truth-telling

Some cultures do not place a great emphasis on informing the patient of the diagnosis, especially when cancer is the diagnosis. American culture rarely used truth-telling especially in medical cases, until 1970s. In American medicine, the principle of informed consent now takes precedence over other ethical values, and patients are usually at least asked whether they want to know the diagnosis.

Online Business Practices

The delivery of diagnosis online leads patients to believe that doctors in some parts of the country are at the direct service of drug companies. Finding diagnosis as convenient as what drug still has patent rights on it. Physicians and drug companies are found to be competing for top ten search engine ranks to lower costs of selling these drugs with little to no patient involvement.

CONFLICTS OF INTEREST

Physicians should not allow a conflict of interest to influence medical judgment. In some cases, conflicts are hard to avoid, and doctors have a responsibility to avoid entering such situations. However, research has shown that conflicts of interests are very common among both academic physicians and in clinical practice.

Referral

For example, doctors who receive income from referring patients for medical diagnostic tests, medicines from pharmacy, etc. have been shown to refer more patients for it.

Commission and **fees splitting** are two major malpractices born due to this referral services.

Treatment of Family Members

Many doctors treat their family members. Doctors who do so must be vigilant not to create conflicts of interest or treat inappropriately.

Sexual Relationships

Sexual relationships between doctors and patients can create ethical conflicts, since sexual consent may conflict with the fiduciary responsibility of the physician. Doctors who enter into sexual relationships with patients face the threats of deregistration and prosecution.

Sexual relationships between physicians and patients' relatives may also be prohibited in some jurisdictions, although this prohibition is highly controversial.

KEY ISSUES OF RESEARCH PUBLICATIONS

In terms of research publications, a number of key issues include:

- **Honesty.** Honesty and integrity is a duty of each author and person, expert-reviewer and member of journal editorial boards.
- **Review process.** The peer-review process contributes to the quality control and it is an essential step to ascertain the standing and originality of the research. The review process should compulsorily involved plagiarism checking using updated software.

- **Ethical standards.** Recent journal editorials presented some experience of unscrupulous activities.
- **Authorship.** Who may claim a right to authorship? In which order should the authors be listed? In India very unlikely, this is questionable. However, it is our moral duties that we could strictly stop these malpractices by refusing these professors burden or interest.
- **Conflict of interest and privacy** are prime important.

22

Informed Consent

LEARNING OBJECTIVES

After reading this chapter student should:
• Be able to define and explain concept of informed consent
• Understand concept of consent assessment
• Know about scope of informed consent
• Know about valid informed consent elements
• Know about concept of patient competency and deception
• Understand values of ethics and informed consent

INTRODUCTION

Informed consent is a process for getting permission before conducting any research activity on a person directly or indirectly or with his records under medical clause.

Informed consent is collected according to guidelines from the fields of medical ethics and research ethics.

An informed consent can be said to have been given based upon a clear appreciation and understanding of the facts, implications, and consequences of an work or action.

To give informed consent, the individual concerned must have adequate reasoning faculties and be in possession of all relevant facts of that research work.

Factors that prevents informed consent being basic intellectual or emotional immaturity, high levels of stress such as PTSD or a severe intellectual disability, severe mental illness, intoxication, severe sleep deprivation, Alzheimer's disease, or being in a coma which leads to impairments to reasoning and judgment.

Whenever such situations are faced by principle investigator, the authorizing person can sign such consent in situations beneficiary to that patient. Example for any trial if there is requirement of children below 2–3 years, that time his parents can be acted as authority signatory. But situation or emergency need is quite important at that time. The principles of bioethics are very important in such situations. Such situations should be handled with to view to independent human being rather than only patient.

Another very important issue is of adequate information. The patient or an individual should provide sufficient and clear information. The serious ethical may arise in such situations when insufficient information is provided to form a reasoned decision.

For practical use various forms or templates necessary for informed consent are available on WHO website.

Consent Assessment

Informed consent can be complex to evaluate, because neither expressions of consent, nor expressions of understanding of implications, necessarily mean that full adult consent was in fact given, nor that full comprehension of relevant issues is internally digested.

Consent may be implied within the usual subtleties of human communication, rather than explicitly negotiated verbally or in writing.

In some cases consent cannot legally be possible, even if the person protests he does indeed understand and wish. There are also structured instruments for evaluating capacity to give informed consent, although no ideal instrument presently exists.

Thus, there is always a degree to which informed consent must be assumed or inferred based upon observation, or knowledge, or legal reliance. This especially is the case in sexual or relational issues. In medical or formal circumstances, explicit agreement by means of signature—normally relied on legally— regardless of actual consent, is the norm. This is the case with certain procedures, such as a "do not resuscitate" directive that a patient signed prior to their illness.

Brief examples of each of the above:

1. A person may be verbally agreed to something from fear, perceived social pressure, or psychological difficulty in asserting true feelings. The person requesting the action may honestly be unaware of this and believe the consent is genuine, and rely on it. Consent is expressed, but not internally given.

2. A person may be claim to understand the implications of some action, as part of consent, but in fact has failed to appreciate the possible consequences fully and may later deny the validity of the consent for this reason. Understanding needed for informed consent is present but is, in fact (through ignorance), not present.

3. A person signs a legal release form for a medical procedure, and later feels he did not really consent. Unless he can show actual misinformation, the release is usually persuasive or conclusive in law, in that the clinician may rely legally upon it for consent. In formal circumstances, a written consent usually legally overrides later denial of informed consent.

Valid Informed Consent Elements

There are three important elements that form valid informed consent, viz. **disclosure, capacity and voluntariness.**

- While **Disclosure** requires the researcher to supply the subject with the information necessary to make an autonomous decision, the investigators must ensure that subjects have adequate comprehension of the information provided. This latter requirement implies that the consent form be written in lay language suited for the comprehension skills of subject population, as well as assessing the level of understanding during the meeting.

- **Capacity** pertains to the ability of the subject to both understand the information provided and form a reasonable judgment based on the potential consequences of his/her decision.

- **Voluntariness** refers to the subject's right to freely exercise his/her decision making without being subjected to external pressure such as coercion, manipulation, or undue influence.

Waiver of the Requirements

Waiver of the consent requirement may be applied in certain situations where no foreseeable harm is expected to result from the study or when permitted by law, federal regulations, or if an ethical review committee has approved the non-disclosure of certain information.

Following are the three important circumstances:

1. Directly benefit subjects.
2. Advance the development of a medical product necessary to the military.
3. Be carried out under all laws and regulations (i.e. Emergency Research Consent Waiver) including those pertinent to the FDA

While informed consent is a basic right and should be carried out effectively, if a patient is incapacitated due to injury or illness, it is still important that patients benefit from emergency experimentation. The Food and Drug Administration (FDA) and the Department of Health and Human Services (DHHS) joined together to create federal guidelines to permit emergency research, without informed consent. However, they can only proceed with the research if they obtain a waiver of informed consent (WIC) or an emergency exception from informed consent (EFIC).

HISTORICAL ASPECTS

"Informed consent" is a technical term first used in a medical malpractice United States court case in 1957.

In tracing its history, some scholars have suggested tracing the history of checking for any of these practices:

1. a patient agrees to a health intervention based on an understanding of it
2. the patient has multiple choices and is not compelled to choose a particular one
3. the consent includes giving permission

These practices are part of what constitutes informed consent, and their history is the history of informed consent. They combine to form the modern concept of informed consent—

which rose in response to particular incidents in modern research. Whereas various cultures in various places practiced informed consent, the modern concept of informed consent was developed by people who drew influence from Western tradition.

Historians cite a series of medical guidelines to trace the history of informed consent in medical practice.

The Hippocratic Oath, a 500 BC Greek text, was the first set of Western writings giving guidelines for the conduct of medical professionals. It advises that physicians conceal most information from patients to give the patients the best care. The rationale is a beneficence model for care—the doctor knows better than the patient, and therefore should direct the patient's care, because the patient is not likely to have better ideas than the doctor.

Thomas Percival was a British physician who published a book called *Medical Ethics* in 1803.

Percival said that patients have a right to truth, but when the physician could provide better treatment by lying or withholding information, he advised that the physician do as he thought best.

Historians cite a series of human subject research experiments to trace the history of informed consent in research.

Medicine in the United States, Australia, and Canada take a more patient-centeric approach to "informed consent."

Obtaining Informed Consents

To capture and manage informed consents, hospital management systems typically use paper-based consent forms which are scanned and stored in a document handling system after obtaining the necessary signatures. Hospital systems and research organizations are adopting an electronic way of capturing informed consents to enable indexing, to improve comprehension, search and retrieval of consent data, thus enhancing the ability to honor to patient intent and identify willing research participants. More recently, Health Sciences South Carolina, a statewide research collaborative focused on transforming healthcare quality, health information systems and patient outcomes, developed an open-source system called Research Permissions Management System (RPMS). RPMS has been released as an open-source application.

PATIENT COMPETENCY

The ability to give informed consent is governed by a general requirement of competency. In common law jurisdictions, adults are presumed competent to consent. This presumption can be rebutted, for instance, in circumstances of mental illness or other incompetence. This may be prescribed in legislation or based on a common-law standard of inability to understand the nature of the procedure. In cases of incompetent adults, a healthcare proxy makes medical decisions. In the absence of a proxy, the medical practitioner is expected to act in the patient's best interests until a proxy can be found.

Deception

Research involving deception is controversial given the requirement for informed consent. Deception typically arises in social psychology, when researching a particular psychological process requires that investigators deceive subjects. For example, in the Milgram experiment, researchers wanted to determine the willingness of participants to obey authority figures despite their personal conscientious objections.

They had authority figures demand that participants deliver what they thought was an electric shock to another researcher. For the study to succeed, it was necessary to deceive the participants so they believed that the subject was a peer and that their electric shocks caused the peer actual pain.

Nonetheless, research involving deception prevents the subject/patient from exercising his/her basic right of autonomous informed decision-making and conflicts with the ethical principle of respect for persons.

The Ethical Principles of Psychologists and Code of Conduct set by the American Psychological Association says that psychologists may not conduct research that includes a deceptive compartment unless they can justify the act by the value and importance of the study's results, and show they could not obtain the results by some other way. Moreover, the research should bear no potential harm to the subject as an outcome of deception, be it physical pain or emotional distress. Finally, the code requires a debriefing session, in which the experimenter tells the subject about the deception, and gives subjects the option of withdrawing their data.

Abortion

In some US states, informed consent laws (sometimes called "right to know" laws) require that a woman seeking an elective abortion receive factual information from the abortion provider about her legal rights, alternatives to abortion (such as adoption), available public and private assistance, and "medical facts" (some of which are disputed—see fetal pain), before the abortion is performed (usually 24 hours in advance of the abortion). Other countries with such laws (e.g. Germany) require that the information giver be properly certified to make sure that no abortion is carried out for the financial gain of the abortion provider and to ensure that the decision to have an abortion is not swayed by any form of incentive.

Informed Consent and Ethics

It is our moral responsibility always to obtain proper informed consent before every act observed with our patient. It is included from simple examination especially of female patients, any medical investigations, any operative either major or minor, etc. The patient should be clearly stated regarding its implications, use, advantages and disadvancetages, risk–benefits, etc. It is prior duty of physician to maintain patient autonomy and justice towards patients. Risk–benefit ratio should be always calculated by doctor on the basis of ethical principles. Patient voluntariness is one of the most important issues which obeys or signifies patient autonomy.

23

Conflict of Interest

LEARNING OBJECTIVES

After reading this chapter student should:

- Be able to define and explain concept of conflict of interest
- Know about the scope of conflict of interest
- Understand basic classification of conflict of interest
- Understand values of ethics in conflict of interest
- Understand competition of interest and conflict of interest

INTRODUCTION

Conflict of interest (COI) is a situation or condition where a research scholar or organization is involved in multiple interests, viz. financial, emotional, or otherwise, one of which could possibly corrupt the motivation, objectives or ethics of the individual or organization.

The presence of a conflict of interest is independent of the occurrence of impropriety. Therefore, a conflict of interest can be discovered and voluntarily defused before any corruption occurs. Most of the time it is observed one of important pillars in any form of corruption either financial or nonfinancial terms. Entry of pharmaceutical competition in market leads incrassates such violations or misconduct concerned with conflict of interest.

Conflict of interest can be simply and broadly divided into two major groups.

1. **Primary conflict of interest** which specifically refers to objectives of concerned research activity, patient protection, research integrity, etc.
2. **Secondary conflict of interest** refers to patient family and relatives concerned with that matter.

It is common observation that in most of the situations conflict of interest is concerned with financial matter.

Though the primary interest is in prime focus, secondary interest has also same importance. Most of researchers are always unaware concern with secondary interest. Though secondary interest is not directly reflected in research work but in most of cases secondary interest is showing most affecting part. The patient relatives always stand front if any misconduct or damage is seen with patient. Hence we as doctors always think regarding secondary interest during our research work and proper documentation is necessary if any uneventful incidence is happened.

Written informed consent is a very important documentation during any such judicial matter and it acts an ethical wall. The details guidelines regarding written informed consent are discussed in Chapter 22 of this textbook.

Conflict of interest may be extended to any institute if that work in such a way that any type of influence may damage personal interest in any way.

Organizational Conflict of Interest

An organizational conflict of interest (OCI) may exist in the same way as described above, for instance, where a corporation provides two types of service to the government and these services conflict (e.g. manufacturing parts and then participating on a selection committee comparing parts manufacturers). Corporations may develop simple or complex systems to mitigate the risk or perceived risk of a conflict of interest. These associated risks can be evaluated by a government agency to determine whether the risks create a substantial advantage to the organization in question over its competition, or will decrease the overall competitiveness of the bidding process.

Conflict of Interest in the healthcare Industry

The conflict of interest nowadays plays a vital role in healthcare industry due to entry of pharmaceutical industry and increment in financial matter. The influence of pharmacy industry either financial ways or any other has major concern with conflict of interest. In 2009 a study found that "a number of academic institutions" do not have clear guidelines for relationships between Institutional Review Boards and industry.

In such contrast to this viewpoint, an article and associated editorial in the New England Journal of Medicine in May 2015 emphasized the importance of pharmaceutical industry—physician interactions for the development of novel treatments, and argued that moral outrage over industry malfeasance had unjustifiably led many to overemphasize the problems created by financial conflicts of interest. The article noted that major healthcare organizations such as National Center for Advancing Translational Sciences of the National Institutes of Health, the President's Council of Advisors on Science and Technology, the World Economic Forum, the Gates Foundation, the Wellcome Trust, and the Food and Drug Administration had encouraged greater interactions between physicians and industry in order to bring greater benefits to patients.

Classification of Conflict of Interest

- **Self-dealing:** It is a concept is which same organizational head is involved in both-sided parties. The very simple example is person who has been selecting for any award or any degree; he is also the same person in selection committee.
- **Outside employment:** In which the interests of one job conflict with another.
- **Nepotism,** in which a spouse, brother or other close relative is employed (or applies for employment) by an individual, or where services are taken from a relative or from a firm controlled by a relative. To avoid nepotism in hiring, many employment applications ask whether the applicant is related to the current employee of the company. This allows refusal if the employed relative has a role in the hiring process. If this is the case, the relative could not be allowed to take any hiring decisions.

- **Gifts from friends** are also considered if that act influence over institutional or organizational decision or any benefit in any means.
- **Pump and dump:** Very simple example is of any stock broker. He always advices his client about same stalks where he already invested. This is one of violations concerned with financial matter.

Other improper acts that are sometimes classified as conflicts of interests are probably better classified elsewhere. **Accepting bribes** can be classified as **corruption**. Use of government or corporate property or assets for personal use is **fraud**. Nor should unauthorized distribution of confidential information, in itself, be considered a conflict of interest.

In research intentionally providing conclusion or highlighted the importance in any way that may favor to some particular association, organization or person is definitely obtained under conflict of interest. As clinicians it is our binding morality to be avoid such consequences. In research ethics this is more clearly explained.

For these improper acts, there is no inherent conflict of **roles** (see above).

COI is sometimes termed **competition of interest** rather than "conflict", emphasizing a connotation of natural competition between valid interests rather than violent conflict with its connotation of victimhood and unfair aggression. Nevertheless, denotatively, there is too much overlap between the terms to make any objective differentiation. Nowadays this form of interest is found increasing frequency due to unawareness and competition in market.

24

Duty to Rescue

LEARNING OBJECTIVES

After reading this chapter student should:

• Be able to define and explain concept of duty to rescue
• Know about laws associated with duty to rescue
• Know about scope of duty to rescue
• Know about legal justifications and duty to rescue
• Understand values of ethics in duty to rescue

INTRODUCTION

A duty to rescue arises where a person creates a hazardous situation. If another person falls into peril because of this hazardous situation, the creator of the hazard—who may not necessarily have been a negligent—has a duty to rescue the individual in peril.

LAWS ASSOCIATED WITH DUTY TO RESCUE

In the common law associated with duty to rescue of most of countries, there is no general duty to come to the rescue of another. Generally, a person cannot be held liable for doing nothing while another person is in peril. However, such a duty may arise in two situations:

• Such a duty may also arise where a "special relationship" exists. For example:

- Parents have a duty to rescue their minor children. This duty also applies to those acting *in loco parentis*, such as schools or babysitters.
- Common carriers have a duty to rescue their patrons.
- Employers have a mandatory obligation to rescue employees, under an implied contract theory.
- In some US jurisdictions, real property owners have a duty to rescue invitees but not trespassers from all reasonably foreseeable dangers on the property. Other jurisdictions, such as California, extend the duty to rescue to all persons who enter upon real property regardless whether they are classified as invitees, social guests or trespassers.
- Spouses have a duty to rescue each other in all US jurisdictions.

Where a duty to rescue arises, the rescuer must generally act with reasonable care, and can be held liable for injuries caused by a reckless rescue attempt. However, many states have limited or removed liability from rescuers in such circumstances, particularly where the rescuer is an emergency worker. Furthermore, the rescuer need not endanger them in conducting the rescue in situations.

Civil Law

Many official civil law systems, which are common in Continental Europe, Latin America and much of Africa express or clarify a far more extensive duty to rescue. The only exclusion is that the person must not endanger his own life or that of others, while providing rescue.

This can mean that if a person finds any person in need of medical help, he must take all reasonable priority steps to seek medical care and render best effort first aid. Commonly, we observe such a situation arises on an event of a traffic accident with prior emergency: other drivers and passers-by must take an action to help the injured without regard to possible personal reasons not to help (e.g. having no time, being in a hurry) or ascertain that help has been requested from officials. In practice, however, almost all cases of compulsory rescue simply require the rescuer to alert the relevant entity (police, fire brigade, ambulance) with a phone call or whatever he can act faster. Because every minute of that person is important during that situation. In such a condition it is our moral responsibility to attain prior help on the basis of humanity.

Ethical Justifications

Legal requirements for a duty to rescue do not pertain in all nations, states, or localities. However, a moral or ethical duty to rescue may exist even where there is no legal duty to rescue. There are such number of potential justifications for such a duty to rescue.

One sort of justification is general and applies regardless of role-related relationships (doctor to patient; firefighter to citizen, etc.). Under this general justification, persons have a duty to rescue other persons in distress by virtue of their common humanity, regardless of the specific skills of the rescuer or the nature of the victim's distress.

Specific arguments for such a duty to rescue include, but are not limited to:

• **The Golden Rule:** Treat others as one would wish to be treated. This considers that all persons would wish to be rescued if they were in distress, and so they should in turn rescue those in distress to the best of their abilities. What counts as distress requiring rescue may, of course, differ from person to person, but being trapped or at risk of drowning are emergent situations which this position assumes all humans would wish to be rescued from.

• **Utilitarianism:** Utilitarianism posits that those actions are right which best maximize happiness and reduce suffering ("maximize the good"). Utilitarian reasoning generally supports acts of rescue which contribute to overall happiness and reduced suffering. Rule utilitarianism would look not just at whether individual acts of rescue maximize the good, but whether certain types of acts do so. It then becomes one's duty to perform those types of actions. Generally, having strangers rescue those in distress maximizes good so long as the rescue attempt does not make things worse, so one has a duty to rescue to the best of their ability as long as doing so will not make things worse.

• **Humanity:** The rules of humanity advise that the essence of morality and right behavior is tending to human relationships. Therefore, virtues (desirable character traits) such as compassion, sympathy, honesty, and fidelity are to be admired and developed. Acting out of compassion and sympathy will often more require rescue where someone is in need. Indeed, it would not be compassionate to ignore someone's need, though the way one fulfills that need may vary. In cases of emergency, rescue would be the most compassionate act compared with allowing a person to remain trapped in rubble.

There are also ethical justifications for role-specific or skill-specific duties of rescue such as those described under the discussion of US Common Law above. Generally, these justifications are rooted in the idea that the *best* rescues, the most effective rescues, are done by those with special skills. Such persons, when available to urgent rescue, are thus even more required to do so ethically than regular persons who might simply make things worse (for a utilitarian, rescue by a skilled professional in a relevant field would maximize the good even better than rescue by a regular stranger). This particular ethical argument makes sense when considering the ability firefighters to get both themselves and victims safely out of a burning building, or of healthcare personnel such as physicians, nurses, physician's assistants, and EMTs to provide medical rescue.

These are some of the ethical justifications for a duty to rescue, and they may hold true for both regular citizens and skilled professionals even in the absence of legal requirements to render aid.

Case Law

In an 1898 case, the New Hampshire Supreme Court unanimously held that after an eight-year-old boy negligently placed his hand in the defendant's machinery, the boy had no right to be rescued by the defendant. Beyond that, the trespassing boy could be held liable for damages to the defendant's machine.

In the 1907 case, People v. Beardsley, Beardsley's mistress, Blanche Burns, passed out after overdosing on morphine. Rather than seek medical attention, Beardsley instead had a friend hide her in the basement, and Burns died a few hours later. Beardsley was tried and convicted of manslaughter for his negligence. However, his conviction was reversed by the Supreme Court of Michigan saying that Beardsley had no legal obligation to her.

These examples should be studied by students and discuss. The output what they sought can improve their vision and mindset regarding urgency and emergency concerned with duty to rescue. From ethical point of view, it is everyone's moral responsibility in view of humanity. Our society always provide credits and goodwill for it.

25

Professionalism and MCI Regulations

"You are in this profession as a calling, not as a business, as a calling which exacts from you at every turn self-sacrifice, devotion, love and tenderness to your fellow-men. Once you get down to a purely business level, your influence is gone and the true light of your life is dimmed."

– **Sir William Osler**

LEARNING OBJECTIVES

After reading this chapter student should:

- Be able to define and explain concept of professionalism
- Know and understand MCI guidelines concerned with professionalism and ethical conduct
- Understand concept of patient confidentiality
- Know about guidelines about devotion of doctor, maintenance of medical records, etc.
- Know about issue of generic drugs and issue of cut practice
- Know about research ethics, professional conduct
- Know about professional misconduct

INTRODUCTION

Professionalism can be defined as dealing with patient with specific trustworthy attitude, behaviors and character which can create patient–physician trust, necessary for good physician with best knowledge and skills required for his cure, along with reflecting moral values.

The concept of professnalisam was explained by a number of experts. Some were explained it on the basis of knowledge while some explain it on the basis of approach, etc. In philosophy it was explained along with ethical approaches and moral values.

It is always topic of debate what are the characteristics and duties of a good physician. How medical colleges seed and can create good doctors for future society? Medical colleges are not just degree certificates factory but are responsible for tomorrow's healthy society and better cure which is the base of a country. Number of medical councils worldwide provides standards for professionalism code. Professionalism is just not maintenance of patient–doctor relationship on business grounds but maintain trust using updated skills, knowledge and attitude with good moral values.

MCI GUIDELINES

The Medical Council of India (MCI) has provided us detailed guidelines regarding applications and conduct in clinical practice. These detail guidelines are available at official website of MCI.

These guidelines included the **professional conduct and ethical approach of doctors.**

According to MCI guidelines, the doctors should maintain **dignity** and **honor** of his profession. The main objective of doctor should be **service to humanity** rather than financial goal like other profession. The society watches us in different eye rather than ordinary view. Hence doctor's approach should be **polite, modest** and he should ready for act anytime when needed. According to MCI, only qualified registered person is allowed for modern medicine practice (allopathy practice) that undergoes detail training as per strict outlines and conduct and qualified.

Patient confidentiality is major and one of the most important measures in medical practice needed for trust of patient. The doctors should maintain confidentiality of patient in every issue and situation. Confidentiality in clinical practice plays a vital role. When patient discloses his private experience with doctor, his investigation reports, any form of diagnosis, any personal information in the interest of societal cause, etc. doctor should bind not to disclose any such records under the provision of medical confidentiality. **Medical confidentiality is an important extended principle of medical bioethics along with informed consent.** Many countries alongwith India has made this a legal provision in their laws.

In medical bioethics, **medical confidentiality** is the most important applied principle after four basic traditional principles suggested by **Tom Beauchamp and James Childress**.

Ethical theories provide many different ways to view confidentiality laws. The doctors should rethink before exposing any information by any means or any third party. He should always first think about his patient duty, patient expectations from him, etc. However, in situations that may hardens others or during some lawful help, doctor should reveals these facts or issues with honest intention and morally without any fear or wrong intension.

Devotion of doctor is another important issue. The devotion should be reflected in every act of doctor. The doctor should always take full measures to update his knowledge and skills necessary for patient care. All conduct of doctors should be on the scientific basis and justifications rather than any violations. According to MCI guidelines the doctor should regularly update his skills. He should attend minimum 30 hours in every five years under clause of continued medical education for skill improvement either through CMEs, Workshops, conferences or research publications, etc. The record of these activities has to submit MCI and then only renewal of registration is possible to doctor. Most of the private clinical practioners are member of Indian Medical Association (IMA). IMA played a very important role for conducting such events, viz. CMEs, Workshops, conferences, etc. IMA always promotes clinical practioners to update clinical skills and knowledge throughout India. When MCI finalized inclusion of bioethics in medical curriculum, IMA immediately voluntarily signed up MOU with MCI and bioethics core curriculum unit, Haifa, Australia. This ceremony was conducted at MUHS, Nashik in May 2015.

MAINTENANCE OF MEDICAL RECORDS

Every doctor should maintain his patient records **at least for 3 years** from the date of commencement of the treatment in a standard proforma laid down by the Medical Council of India. If any request is made for medical records either by patients/authorised attendant or legal authorities involved, the same may be duly acknowledged and documents shall be issued **within the period of 72 hours.**

A Registered medical practitioner should maintain a Register of Medical Certificates giving full details of certificates issued to his patient. When issuing a medical certificate he should always enter the identification marks of the patient and keep a copy of the certificate. He should not omit to record the signature and/or thumb mark, address and at least one identification mark of the patient on the medical certificates or report. These certificates should be issued in specified proforma declared by MCI.

Issue of Generic Drugs

As far as possible every doctor should mention generic drugs name over patient prescription. Use of rational drug prescription is a major issue in today's clinical practice. The cost of generic drug is obviously very low as compare to branded drugs. In India, a few patients can afford such costly treatment. Alongwith cost factors, it is observed and proved fact that the effects of generic drugs are almost same as branded drugs. But due to lobbing of private pharma companies among private clinicians, these promote branded drugs. Hence practices of generic drugs laid behind since few years back. Nowadays MCI as well as government took up necessary promising steps for the promotion of generic drugs.

Issue of Payment or Doctor's Charges

According MCI guidelines payment or charges towards doctors should never be issue leading to conflict of interest while offering services to patient. The doctor should be always offering the patient what he could offer best at that situation rather than thinking pay issue.

A doctor should state his charges before rendering service and not after the operation or treatment is under way. Remuneration received for such services should be in the form and amount specifically announced to the patient at the time the service is rendered. It is unethical to enter into a contract of "no cure no payment". Physician rendering service on behalf of the state shall refrain from anticipating or accepting any consideration.

Clinical Practice and Laws

The doctor should observe laws in our country while in clinical practice. He should cautious concern with laws applicable in issue of public health betterment.

Doctor should observe the provisions of the State Acts like Drugs and Cosmetics Act, 1940; Pharmacy Act, 1948; Narcotic Drugs and Psychotropic Substances Act, 1985; Medical Termination of Pregnancy Act, 1971; Transplantation of Human Organ Act, 1994; Mental Health Act, 1987; Environmental Protection Act, 1986; Prenatal Sex Determination Test Act, 1994; Drugs and Magic Remedies (Objectionable Advertisement) Act, 1954; Persons with Disabilities (Equal Opportunities and Full Participation) Act, 1995 and Bio-Medical Waste (Management and Handling) Rules, 1998 and such other Acts, Rules, Regulations made by the Central/State Governments or local Administrative Bodies or any other relevant act relating to the protection and promotion of public health (**as per MCI guidelines**).

Duties of Doctor Towards His Patient

Even if doctor is not bound to cure or treat every patient asks for his services but he should be ready to respond to the calls of the **sick and the injured first**.

Patience and delicacy should characterize the doctor. Confidences concerning individual or domestic life entrusted by patients to a physician and defects in the disposition or character of patients observed during medical attendance should never be revealed unless their revelation is required by the laws of the State. Sometimes, however, a physician must determine whether his duty to society requires him to employ knowledge, obtained through confidence as a physician, to protect a healthy person against a communicable disease to which he is about to be exposed. In such instance, the physician should act as he would wish another to act toward one of his own family like circumstances. (as per MCI guidelines).

When a doctor is **called for consultation**, he should not normally take charges for that case. He should not criticize the referring doctor. He should discuss the diagnosis treatment plan with the referring doctor.

ADVERTISEMENTS

Lawfully, there is ban over the advertisements done by doctors with statement with their charges, etc. in newspapers or any electronic media. This is also ethically not correct.

However, some exemptions are mentioned by MCI:

1. On starting practice.
2. On change of type of practice.
3. On changing address.
4. On temporary absence from duty.
5. On resumption of another practice.
6. On succeeding to another practice.
7. Public declaration of charges.

ISSUE OF CUT PRACTICE

Nowadays issue of cut practice or charges spitting by doctor is found more than previous days. It is our sole responsibility to be strict against such misconduct.

As per MCI Guidelines

MCI guidelines clause numbers 6.4.1 and 6.4.2: 6.4.1—A physician shall not give, solicit, or receive nor shall he offer to give solicit or receive, any gift, gratuity, commission or bonus in consideration of or return for the referring, recommending or procuring of any patient for medical, surgical or other treatment. A physician shall not directly or indirectly, participate in or be a party to act of division, transference, assignment, subordination, rebating, splitting or refunding of any fee for medical, surgical or other treatment. 6.4.2—Provisions of para **6.4.1** shall apply with equal force to the referring, recommending or procuring by a physician or any person, specimen or material for diagnostic purposes or other study / work. Nothing in this section, however, shall prohibit payment of salaries by a qualified physician to other duly qualified person rendering medical care under his supervision.

Euthanasia

Euthanasia or **mercy killing** is one of the most controversial issues in medical practice worldwide scenario.

According to MCI, practice of euthanasia should constitute unethical conduct. However, on specific situation, the question of withdrawing supporting devices to sustain cardio-pulmonary function even after brain death shall be decided only by a team of doctors and not merely by treating physician alone. A team of doctors shall declare withdrawal of support system. Such team shall consist of the doctor in charge of the patient, Chief Medical Officer/Medical Officer in charge of the hospital and a doctor nominated by in-charge of the hospital from the hospital staff or in accordance with the provisions of the Transplantation of Human Organ Act, 1994.

In view of the inconsistent opinions observed in Aruna Shanbaug case by court and also considering the important question of law involved which required to be reflected in the light of social, legal, medical and constitutional perspective, it becomes an important need to have a clear enunciation of law.

Elsewhere in the world active euthanasia is almost always illegal. The legal status of passive euthanasia, on the other hand, including the withdrawal of nutrition or water, varies across the nations of the world. As India had no law about euthanasia, the Supreme Court's guidelines are law until and unless our Parliament passes legislation.

Human Rights

The fundamental rights which describe the specific standards, principles or norms of human behavior and are regularly protected as legal rights, irrespective of nation, location, religion or any other status are known as **human rights.** These rights are applicable for everyone irrespective of individual. If these are applicable to all of us, it is our duty to obey their regulations and always act everyday to prevent or damages rights of others. Nowadays worldwide human rights became one strong movement. Constitution of India provides for fundamental rights, which include freedom of religion, freedom of speech, freedom of movement within the country and abroad, etc. According to MCI, the doctor should not torture or act in any means that may lead to violation of human rights.

MCI guidelines also discussed issue concerned with **research ethics, professional conduct,** etc. in detail.

Fundamental Ethical Issues and Unnecessary Surgical Procedures

Performing unnecessary surgical procedures is inconsistent with ethical practice because all surgical procedures bear some degree of risk. It is a major betrayal of the surgeon's paramount obligation to place the patient's best interests first in therapeutic decisions. Every year millions of patients go under knife, but many of them are enduring great pain and shelling out thousands and dollars for surgeries they don't really need. The estimated figure for the unnecessary surgical operations varies from 30 to 70%. There are some healthcare providers who perform surgeries simply because profit. It is surgeon's moral responsibility to do best for patient and think whether it is appropriate for a particular patient or not. Medical justification and desire of patient and qualification of surgeon for that operative is another important ethical issue. It is not justifiable to do unnecessary surgical operations only for the sake of benefits to hospitals. According to fundamental code of ethics always consider first the well-being of the patient. The patient being treated at the time must be the physician's primary concern. Informed consent provides adequate information about the risks, benefits, and alternatives before any surgery. Performing unnecessary surgery violates rules of fundamental code of ethics. It may be a basis for malpractice liability or tort actions for fraud and battery. It may be difficult to prove which cases are unnecessary. But unnecessary surgery is that which is clearly medically unjustifiable when the risks and costs exceed the likely therapeutic benefits to the patient based on the patient's lifestyle requirements.

Professional Misconduct

Any violation or deviation in such conduct declared by MCI in clinical practice is considered as professional misconduct. The punishment and necessary disciplinary action can be obtained by MCI in such cases of misconduct by any doctor. The detail guidelines for necessary steps are mentioned by Medical Council of India on their official website.

Professionalism and Ethics

Along with professional approach of doctors nowadays it is linked with ethics and philosophy towards its foundation. Actually in real sense this approach was observed since back from Hippocrates. But nowadays its urgent need for us. To maintain our own profession as Nobel, it is our responsibility to maintain its values and tradition in modern world. Every aspect of life cannot be judged on the basis of money and time. Medical practice is the single most profession in the world to which people faith alongside God.

In modern era medical profession has been severely challenged by changing social forces and situations. However, it is our responsibility to maintain the dignity and value of our profession. The foundation of ethics would definitely can change our mindset. The burning issues concerns with fees splitting, malpractice, cut practice, unnecessary operatives, etc. would be definitely decreasing with of ethics teaching in medical curriculum. Medical bioethics is based on the framework postulated by **Tom Beauchamp and James Childress**. It is based on four fundamental principles which are to be judged against each other.

In applying and advancing scientific knowledge, medical practice and associated technologies, human vulnerability should be taken into account. Individuals and groups of special vulnerability should be protected and the personal integrity of such individuals respected.

In conclusion, the **autonomy** is the right provided to the patient, simultaneously doctor has to obey principles of **beneficence** and **non-maleficence** that means he has to provide best treatment to his patient and see his patient should not suffer from any harm during the treatment. The base of medical ethics stands on this conclusion which extends with provision of **justice**. Patient justice is the first duty of any doctor.

Tom Beauchamp and James Childress framed their model of medical bioethics on this concept and proposed these four parameters as **basic fundamental principles of medical bioethics**.

The practice of medicine is not a business and can never be one... Our fellow creatures cannot be dealt with as a man deals in corn and coal; the human heart by which we live must control our professional relations.

— **Sir William Osler**

26

The Right to Information (RTI) Act of India

LEARNING OBJECTIVES

After reading this chapter student should:

• Be able to define and explain concept of RTI Act of India
• Know about scope of RTI Act
• Know about process and charges of RTI Act of India
• Know about benefits of RTI Act of India
• Know about Freedom of Information Act 2002

INTRODUCTION

The Right to Information (RTI) Act is an act of the Parliament of India replaces the Freedom of Information Act, 2002 which was compulsorily applies to all States and Union Territories of India except Jammu and Kashmir.

Under the provisions of the Act, any citizen of India may request any information from a "public authority" which is required to mandatorily reply expeditiously or within 30 days.

The Act requires every public authority to make computerize their records for wide and quick dissemination and to proactively certain categories of information so that the citizens need minimum recourse to request for information formally. This law was passed by Parliament on 15 June 2005 and came fully into force on 12 October 2005. The first application under this Act was given to a Pune police station in Maharashtra.

Information disclosure in India was restricted by the Official Secrets Act 1923 and various other special laws, which the new RTI Act relaxes. It protects a fundamental right of citizens.

Famous social worker **Mr Anna Hajare** from Ralegan Siddhi, Maharashtra opened a huge movement against state and central government for implementing this act urgently for the benefits of every citizen of India.

Finally the Act was passed under the name of **The Right to Information Act** or very popularly known as **RTI Act** in media and population.

FREEDOM OF INFORMATION ACT 2002

The Central Government appointed a working group under HD Shourie and assigned it the task of drafting legislation. The Shourie draft, was the basis for the Freedom of Information Bill, 2000 which eventually became law under the Freedom of Information Act, 2002. This Act was severely criticized for permitting too many exemptions, not only under the standard grounds of national security and sovereignty, but also for requests that would involve "disproportionate diversion of the resources of a public authority". There was no upper limit on the charges that could be levied.

STATE-LEVEL RTI ACTS

The state-level RTI Acts were first successfully enacted by the state governments of Tamil Nadu (1997), Goa (1997), Rajasthan (2000), Delhi (2001), Maharashtra (2002), Assam(2002), Madhya Pradesh (2003), Jammu and Kashmir (2004), and Haryana (2005), Andhra Pradesh (2005).

The RTI Act cover all constitutional authorities, including the executive, legislature and judiciary; any institution or body established or constituted by an Act of Parliament or a state legislature. It is also defined in the Act that bodies or authorities established or constituted by order or notification of appropriate government including bodies "owned, controlled or substantially financed" by government, or non-government organizations "substantially financed, directly or indirectly by funds" provided by the government are also covered in the Act.

Private bodies

Private bodies are not within the Act's ambit directly. In a decision of Sarbajit Roy versus Delhi Electricity Regulatory

Commission, the Central Information Commission also reaffirmed that privatised public utility companies continue to be within the RTI Act—their privatisation not withstanding.

Political parties

The Central Information Commission (CIC), consisting of Satyanand Mishra, ML Sharma and Annapurna Dixit, has held that the political parties are public authorities and are answerable to citizens under the RTI Act.

PROCESS OF RTI

The RTI process involves reactive (as opposed to proactive) disclosure of information by the authorities. An RTI written submitted request initiates the process.

Each authority covered by the RTI Act must appoint their Public Information Officer (PIO). Any person may submit a written request to the PIO for information. It is the PIO's obligation to provide information to citizens of India who request information under the Act. If the request pertains to another public authority (in whole or part), it is the PIO's responsibility to transfer/forward the concerned portions of the request to a PIO of the other authority within 5 working days. In addition, every public authority is required to designate Assistant Public Information Officers (APIOs) to receive RTI requests and appeals for forwarding to the PIOs of their public authority. The applicant is required to disclose his name and contact particulars but not any other reasons or justification for seeking information.

The Central Information Commission (CIC) acts upon complaints from those individuals who have not been able to submit information requests to a Central Public Information Officer or State Public Information Officer due to either the officer not having been appointed, or because the respective Central Assistant Public Information Officer or State Assistant Public Information Officer refused to receive the application for information.

The Act specifies time limits for replying to the request.

• If the request has been made to the PIO, the reply is to be given within 30 days of receipt.

- If the request has been made to an APIO, the reply is to be given within 35 days of receipt.
- If the PIO transfers the request to another public authority (better concerned with the information requested), the time allowed to reply is 30 days but computed from the day after it is received by the PIO of the transferee authority.
- Information concerning corruption and Human Rights violations by scheduled Security agencies (those listed in the Second Schedule to the Act) is to be provided within 45 days but with the prior approval of the Central Information Commission.
- However, if life or liberty of any person is involved, the PIO is expected to reply within 48 hours.

Since the information is to be paid for, the reply of the PIO is necessarily limited to either denying the request (in whole or part) and/or providing a computation of "further fees". The time between the reply of the PIO and the time taken to deposit the further fees for information is excluded from the time allowed. If information is not provided within this period, it is treated as deemed refusal. Refusal with or without reasons may be ground for appeal or complaint. Further, information not provided in the times prescribed is to be provided free of charge. Appeal processes are also defined.

Charges

A citizen who wish to seek some information from a public authority is required to send, along with the application, a demand draft or a bankers cheque or an Indian Postal Order of ₹ 10/- (Rupees ten) payable to the Accounts Officer of the public authority as fee prescribed for seeking information.

The applicant may also be required to pay further fee towards the cost of providing the information, details of which shall be intimated to the applicant by the PIO as prescribed by the **RTI Act Exclusions.**

Central Intelligence and Security agencies specified in the Second Schedule like IB, Directorate General of Income tax (Investigation), RAW, Central Bureau of Investigation (CBI), Directorate of Revenue Intelligence, Central Economic Intelligence Bureau, Directorate of Enforcement, Narcotics

Control Bureau, Aviation Research Centre, Special Frontier Force, BSF, CRPF, ITBP, CISF, NSG, Assam Rifles, Special Service Bureau, Special Branch (CID), Andaman and Nicobar, The Crime Branch-CID-CB, Dadra and Nagar Haveli and Special Branch, Lakshadweep Police. Agencies specified by the State Governments through a Notification will also be excluded. The exclusion, however, is not absolute and these organizations have an obligation to provide information pertaining to allegations of corruption and human rights violations. Further, information relating to allegations of human rights violation could be given but only with the approval of the Central or State Information Commission.

INFORMATION EXCLUSIONS

The following is exempt from disclosure under Section 8 of the Act:

- Information, disclosure of which would prejudicially affect the sovereignty and integrity of India, the security, "strategic, scientific or economic" interests of the state, relation with foreign state or lead to incitement of an offense;
- Information which has been expressly forbidden to be published by any court of law or tribunal or the disclosure of which may constitute contempt of court;
- Information, the disclosure of which would cause a breach of privilege of Parliament or the State Legislature;
- Information including commercial confidence, trade secrets or intellectual property, the disclosure of which would harm the competitive position of a third party, unless the competent authority is satisfied that larger public interest warrants the disclosure of such information;
- Information available to a person in his fiduciary relationship, unless the competent authority is satisfied that the larger public interest warrants the disclosure of such information;
- Information received in confidence from foreign government, etc.
- Information, the disclosure of which can endanger the life or physical safety of any person or identify the source of

information or assistance given in confidence for law enforcement or security purposes;

• Information which can impede the process of investigation or apprehension or prosecution of offenders;

• Cabinet papers including records of deliberations of the Council of Ministers, Secretaries and other officers;

• Information which is related to personal information, the disclosure of which has no relationship to any public activity or interest, or which would cause unwarranted invasion of the privacy of the individual (but it is also provided that the information which cannot be denied to the Parliament or a State Legislature shall not be denied by this exemption).

Notwithstanding any of the exemptions listed above, a public authority may allow access to information, if public interest in disclosure outweighs the harm to the protected interests. However, this does not apply to disclosure of "trade or commercial secrets protected by law ".

27

Hippocratic Oath

LEARNING OBJECTIVES

After reading this chapter student should:

- Be able to explain the concept of Hippocratic oath and its elements
- Know about historical aspects of Hippocratic oath

INTRODUCTION

The **Hippocratic oath** is an oath officially taken by every clinician which is written by Hippocrates , known as Father of medicine, in Ionic Greek, in the late 5th Century BCE.

In its original form, it requires a new physician to swear, by a number of healing Gods, to uphold specific ethical standards. In every country the forms may be seen variable though content is continued and same. It is updated or revised every time along with years. Nowadays what we use is known as modern version of Hippocratic oath.

Historically there is seen conflict who actually wrote it originally. Some experts of history says that it was written by one student of Hippocrates while some says that it may be written by Pythagoreans . How it was named Hippocratic oath is also issue of debate.

Oath is an ideal way to promise ethical behavior. In every religion there is stated importance of oath.

ORIGINAL VERSION OF HIPPOCRATIC OATH

This is the original version of the Hippocratic Oath:

"I swear by Apollo the physician, and Aesculapius the surgeon, likewise Hygeia and Panacea, and call all the Gods and Goddesses to witness, that I will observe and keep this underwritten oath, to the utmost of my power and judgment.

I will reverence my master who taught me the art. Equally with my parents, will I allow him things necessary for his support, and will consider his sons as brothers. I will teach them my art without reward or agreement; and I will impart all my acquirement, instructions, and whatever I know, to my master's children, as to my own; and likewise to all my pupils, who shall bind and tie themselves by a professional oath, but to none else.

With regard to healing the sick, I will devise and order for them the best diet, according to my judgment and means; and I will take care that they suffer no hurt or damage.

Nor shall any man's entreaty prevail upon me to administer poison to anyone; neither will I counsel any man to do so. Moreover, I will give no sort of medicine to any pregnant woman, with a view to destroy the child.

Further, I will comport myself and use my knowledge in a godly manner.

I will not cut for the stone, but will commit that affair entirely to the surgeons.

Whatsoever house I may enter, my visit shall be for the convenience and advantage of the patient; and I will willingly refrain from doing any injury or wrong from falsehood, and (in an especial manner) from acts of an amorous nature, whatever may be the rank of those who it may be my duty to cure, whether mistress or servant, bond or free.

Whatever, in the course of my practice, I may see or hear (even when not invited), whatever I may happen to obtain knowledge of, if it be not proper to repeat it, I will keep sacred and secret within my own breast.

If I faithfully observe this oath, may I thrive and prosper in my fortune and profession, and live in the estimation of posterity; or on breach thereof, may the reverse be my fate!"

Modern Version of Hippocratic Oath

"I swear to fulfill, to the best of my ability and judgment, this covenant:

I will respect the hard-won scientific gains of those physicians in whose steps I walk, and gladly share such knowledge as is mine with those who are to follow. I will apply, for the benefit of the sick, all measures which are required, avoiding those twin traps of overtreatment and therapeutic nihilism. I will remember that there is art to medicine as well as science, and that warmth, sympathy, and understanding may outweigh the surgeon's knife or the chemist's drug. I will not be ashamed to say "I know not," nor will I fail to call in my colleagues when the skills of another are needed for a patient's recovery. I will respect the privacy of my patients, for their problems are not disclosed to me that the world may know. Most especially must I tread with care in matters of life and death. If it is given me to save a life, all thanks. But it may also be within my power to take a life; this awesome responsibility must be faced with great humbleness and awareness of my own frailty. Above all, I must not play at God. I will remember that I do not treat a fever chart, a cancerous growth, but a sick human being, whose illness may affect the person's family and economic stability. My responsibility includes these related problems, if I am to care adequately for the sick. I will prevent disease whenever I can, for prevention is preferable to cure. I will remember that I remain a member of society, with special obligations to all my fellow human beings, those sound of mind and body as well as the infirm. If I do not violate this oath, may I enjoy life and art, respected while I live and remembered with affection thereafter. May I always act so as to preserve the finest traditions of my calling and may I long experience the joy of healing those who seek my help."

This modern version is written by Louis Lasagna, Academic Dean of the School of Medicine at Tufts University in 1964 which is nowadays used in many medical colleges and university across the globe.

Modern Use and Relevance

Number of times this oath is modified or revised. In 1948 it was revised by World Medical Association known as **Declaration of Geneva.**

Immediately after second world war World Medical Association (WMA) take responsibility of setting up ethics and ethical practices in medical sector worldwide. At that time oath was given to every medical graduate at time end of his graduation and before issuing him degree in medical field.

In 1960s, the Hippocratic Oath was changed to require "utmost respect for human life from its beginning", making it a more secular obligation, not to be taken in the presence of God, but before other people. When the Oath was revised in 1964 by Louis Lasagna at Tufts University, the prayer part was omitted, and that version has been widely accepted and is still in use today by most of medical colleges and universities across the globe.

In the United States, the majority of osteopathic medical schools use the Osteopathic Oath in place of or in addition to the Hippocratic Oath. The Osteopathic Oath was first used in 1938, and the current version has been in use since 1954.

In a 1989 survey of 126 US medical schools, only three reported use of the original oath, while thirty-three used the Declaration of Geneva, sixty-seven used a modified Hippocratic Oath, four used the Oath of Maimonides, one used a covenant, eight used another oath, one used an unknown oath, and two did not use any kind of oath. Seven medical schools did not reply to the survey.

In a 2000 survey of US medical colleges and universities, all of the then extent medical schools administered some type of profession oath. Among schools of modern medicine, sixty-two of 122 used the Hippocratic Oath, or a modified version of it. The other sixty schools used the original or modified Declaration of Geneva, Oath of Maimonides, or an oath authored by students and or faculty. All nineteen osteopathic schools used the Osteopathic Oath.

In France, it is common for new medical graduates to sign a written oath.

In 1991, José High was set to be executed in Georgia, United States. The execution team could not gain access to Jose High's vein due to extreme drug use from his past. The execution team brought in a doctor who had critical care training and was an expert at finding deep veins in the human body. Once the doctor was hired for the sole reason of inserting an IV, the doctor at that point became part of the execution team.

Up until this point, doctors would not take part in placing an IV or administering the drugs, but were only there to pronounce the death of the inmate. The execution happened without incident. However, a group of doctors sued the Georgia State Medical Board for not disciplining the doctor, stating that he violated federal law and broke the Hippocratic Oath (although the Hippocratic oath is not legally binding). In response, the Georgia legislature passed laws protecting doctors who take part in lethal injections from civil and criminal prosecution.

[**Note:** To avoid changes in meaning of sentence or message to medical students, original version and Modern version of Hippocratic Oath is downloaded on 28 June 2015 from www.wikipedia.com]

28

Attitude and Communication

LEARNING OBJECTIVES

After reading this chapter the student should:

- Understand the Bloom's taxonomy and attitude in clinical practice.
- Understand the relationship between positive attitude and effective communication
- Understand the basic facts concerned with effective communication approach
- Understand factors influencing communication and guidelines for effective communication
- Understand factors influencing positive attitude and effective communication
- Understand methods to overcome barriers of communication
- Understand interpersonal relationship and communication in clinical practice
- Understand the role and responsibilities of the physician in society.
- Understand patients behavior and expectations from doctor
- Understand ideal doctor–patient relationship components
- Understand patients rights
- Understand ethical approach in patient communication

INTRODUCTION

Physician is not only person concerned with curative approach but also accountable for preventive care, holistic care, promotive and palliative care of community. In other words, in extent of order the medical graduate is not just a doctor but he is also leader of society, communicator as well as counselor, lifelong learner and professional who is committed for the best, ethical, responsive and accountable to our society. Good communication skills has a vital role in improving the doctor–patient relationship and leads to improved patient compliance, satisfaction with care and benefits to physical and mental health of patients. Effective communication with patients would definitely leads positive impact on overall doctors professional skills.

Our attitudes has three main components, affective (the way we feel), cognitive (the way we think) and behavioral (the way we act) towards a particular entity. Hence it is necessary to seed yourself the basic attitude and communication competencies as medical professional from your early years of learning. Our knowledge may not change our attitude but our experience will definitely change our attitude. Positive thinking and responsiveness towards others are the key area of thinking towards creating positive attitude.

BLOOM'S TAXONOMY AND ATTITUDE

The relationship between positive attitudes toward effective communication skills training during study period and the effective learning of these skills is consistent with several models of learning, most notably Bloom's (1956) taxonomy of educational objectives. On the basis of Bloom taxonomy, he classified medical learning into three major domains, viz. **knowledge (cognition), skills (psychomotor skills) and attitude (affect).** While there has been some interest in applying Bloom's taxonomy to medical student educational content. These studies have primarily focused on the cognitive and psychomotor dimensions of Bloom's taxonomy as opposed to the affective domain. Moreover, these studies have not clearly specify the relationships between affective aspects of the taxonomy, such as medical student attitudes toward communication skills training, on learning outcomes such as knowledge of appropriate medical communication behavior, perceived importance of communication skills, or self-assessments of confidence in communicating with patients.

However, Bloom's taxonomy serves as a useful theoretical framework for studying medical student attitudes towards communication skills training. Repeated seeding of thoughts in classrooms, clinics, etc. and regular measurements of perception-based attitude scale will be one effective statistically proven parameter for the output of effective communication and future competent doctor for our society.

Positive thinking and attitude alway lead towards effective communication skills.

Communication

It is a process involving transfer of information and thoughts or content to another person.

In clinical scenario communication plays a vital role when dealing with patients. Effective communication is always considering good health indicator of concerned doctor in community. Majority of recent trends or misconducts is basically due to a lack of good communication.

Watzlawick et al's Four Basic Principles of Communication

Watzlawick et al stated four basic principles of communication in daily practices which are applicable to every communication. These are stated as follows:

1. One cannot communicate.
2. Every communication has a content and relationship aspect.
3. As a result of series of communications formed series of interchanges.
4. All communication relationships are either symmetrical or complementary.

However, it is interesting to say that how our communication can become more effective. **American Management Association (AMA)** has stated essentials of good communication which are applicable in our daily practices and can boost effective communication. These are popularly known as **"Ten commands of good communication"**.

These are stated as follows:

1. Clarifies ideas before your communication
2. Examine the true purposes of your communication

3. Take entire environment into consideration

4. Whenever valuable or required advice, obtain it from others

5. Beware of the overtones.

6. Whenever possible to you, just convey useful information

7. Follow up on every communication

8. Communicate with the future as well as present in your mind set

9. Always supports your words with deeds

10. Always be a good listener

These ten commands will definitely be fruitful and makes our daily communication with our patients more effective with improving our positive attitude.

When we think in detail, communication can be analyzed simply using mnemonics seven Cs of communication. Once we understands these basic foundations which makes our communication good, it can be visibly enters in our daily approaches with our patients.

Seven Cs of Communication

1. Credibility:

2. Content

3. Context

4. Channels

5. Clarity

6. Capability

7. Consistency

Factors Influencing Communication

There are a large number of factors which can influence our communication. Herewith we listed factors which affect our communication with patients.

1. Situational factors—stress, fear, anxiety, fatigue, inability of mind to listen or act.

2. Psychological factors

3. Social factors

4. Environmental factors, etc.

Guidelines for Effective Communication

1. Always be a good listener.
2. Always avoid extremes in speaking in any matter. This is one of the most important issues which lead to become major obstacle in any misconduct or incidence that hampers our act.
3. Clarify ideas in gentle manner.
4. Feedback to every communication.
5. Not to talk and talk.
6. Understand purpose of communication.
7. Should know your audience.
8. Avoid words which have vague meanings.

Barriers of Effective Communication in Clinical Practice

Following is a list of barriers of effective communication in clinical practice setup.

1. Superiority barrier
2. To maintain authority or ownership
3. Self satisfaction
4. Overloaded burden of work
5. Environmental disturbances
6. Physical ill health
7. Cross cultural barriers
8. Perception barriers
9. Interpersonal barriers
10. Facilities barriers—inadequate facilities for doctors
11. Status and position barriers
12. Unclarity of assumption

Methods to Overcome Barriers of Communication

1. Always be a good and active listener.
2. Use appropriate words.
3. Clarity in your speech and act.
4. Know the receivers or your patient.
5. Good interpersonal relationship built

6. Proper actions and deeds.

7. Feedback of your communication and suitable act.

Functions of Communication in Clinical Practice

1. Instruct your patient

2. Inform your patient

3. Influence your patient

4. Patient interview or history taking

5. Patient directives in treatment plan of action

6. Decision making with patients

7. Patient orientation with fact or situation

8. Patient education or instructions, etc.

Interpersonal Relationship and Communication in Clinical Practice

Communication basically depends upon interpersonal relationships among doctors and patients. Various factors which can influence interpersonal relations of doctor–patient can be summarized herewith.

1. Trust of patient

2. Patient empathy

3. Patient value or equalities

4. Caring approach of doctor

5. Patient autonomy

Guidelines of Patient-oriented Communication and Attitude of Doctor

It is physician's first priority that his every communication with patients should be in such a way that patient must able to trust on doctor. To create trust it is doctor's responsibility to show respect for human life, patients every concern, maintain patient autonomy, respect for patients rights, etc. On this basis the patient's every visit to clinic of doctor should be construct in such a way that:

1. It would build doctor–patient relations more trustworthy.

2. Gathering information from doctor in ethical manner.

3. Understands patient's requirements and perspectives.

4. Information sharing and options.

5. Understands and communicate with patient in such a wayes that doctor understands his pain, emergency, responsibility and priority in treatment plan.

With this view in mind, doctor should be competent to communicate with patient:

1. He can eliciting patients main problems and perception of these as well as emotional and societal impact of patients ill health on him, over his family and relatives as a whole.

2. Doctor can tailoring information to need based of patient.

3. Eliciting patient's reactions to information provided in visit.

4. Assessing patient's wish participation concern in treatment plan implementation.

5. Discussion treatment option with patient, hence maintain patient autonomy.

   Finally it is core need to correlate positive attitude towards effective communication skills. Caring and sharing visible approach of doctor reflects his attitude. Caring approach is outlined by doctor's respect and sensitivity towards patient's emotions and experiences while sharing approach is outlined by doctor's willingness to share medical information. This is especially true and highly observed in breaking bad news and in emergency situations. Both these approaches in combination reflect doctor's overall attitude. To overcome situations and to be a best doctor, positive attitude plays vital role and reflects in communication with patients.

   In conclusion to improve the effective communication with positive attitude:

   • The doctor's caring and sharing approach plays vital role

   • The doctor understands ability to patients

   • The doctor understands patient emergency and autonomy

   • The doctor respects and approach towards patient autonomy

   • The doctor's respects towards patient's cultural values

   • The doctor's behavior and act during patient visit and following treatment course.

Strategies to facilitate effective communication by doctors
1. Be always good and active listener
2. Always share your observations in clinical practice
3. Sharing hope with your patient
4. Sharing emotions with your patient
5. Sharing reality with your patient
6. Provide proper information to your patient
7. Always ask relevant questions to your patient
8. Share humor with your patient
9. Be remember, using silence may sometime speak your act.
10. Clarities in your ideas, discussion with your patient
11. The severity of patient illness may affect doctors approach.
12. Proper summation of the situation or fact to patient

Most of times doctors have to act as counselor towards patient. The doctor should ideally always good counselor with patient.

Characteristics of Good Counselors
1. Understanding
2. Sympathetic attitude
3. Friendliness
4. Kindness
5. Calmness
6. Fairness in information discussion
7. Tactful talk
8. Sincerity of efforts and plan of action
9. Patience
10. Stability
11. Sense of humor
12. Tolerance
13. Objectivity
14. Clarity of concept
15. Broadmindedness approach
16. Poise
17. Societal intelligence

ROLE AND RESPONSIBILITIES OF PHYSICIAN IN COMMUNITY

The doctors in Indian scenario are always considering in places of God as second person after God. Hence in such Nobel profession every patient expects best from doctor's so that he could cure or saves from life threatening. Our cultural values also boost these situations. Hence doctors himself should be responsive towards society and community. As a responsible it is his moral duty to upgrade his knowledge throughout lifetime and implement better technologies in day-to-day practices so that his patient will receives best from doctors. This is prime and most important responsibility of every doctor. Empathy in patient encounter is second most important issue concerned with emergency.

Ideal Doctor–patient Relationship Components

- **Patient confidentiality:** Confidentiality in clinical practice plays a vital role. When patient discloses his private experience with doctor, his investigation reports, his any form of diagnosis, his any personal information in interest of societal cause etc, doctors should bind not to disclose any such records under the provision of medical confidentiality. *Medical confidentiality is an important extended principle of medical bioethics along with informed consent.* Many countries alongwith India has made this a legal provision in their laws.

- **Ensure patient understands:** It is second most important issue concerned with maintaining good doctor–patient relationships. The good doctor–patient relations can only be formed on the basis of patient trust. The doctor should always obey his communication in every situation, henceforth patient understands every step in treatment protocol, etc.

- **Devotion** of doctor is another important issue. The devotion should be reflected in every act of doctor. The doctor should always take full measures to update his knowledge and skills necessary for patient care. All conduct of doctors should be on the scientific basis and justifications rather than any violations.

- **Patience and delicacy** should characterize the doctor. Confidences concerning individual or domestic life entrusted by patients to a physician and defects in the disposition or character of patients observed during medical attendance should never be revealed unless their revelation is required by the laws of the State. Sometimes, however, a physician must determine whether his duty to society requires him to employ knowledge, obtained through confidence as a physician, to protect a healthy person against a communicable disease to which he is about to be exposed.

- **Responding to patient questions:** The doctors should be responsive towards every query placed by his patient.
  - **Never hide anything from patient**
  - **Listening of the patients**
  - **Non-discrimination of patients**
  - **Patient support by every way**
- **Patient Respect:** The principles of autonomy are based on the right of individuals to self-determination. Nowadays clinical practice is shifted more towards patient oriented, the value of autonomy increased. Respect for autonomy is the basis for informed consent and advance directives. By autonomy it is patient right what he wants? Refusal to treatment or any investigations or any surgical procedure is sole autonomy of any patient.
- **Maintenance of ethical conduct**
- **Beneficence:** The action or act that promotes well-being of others is known as beneficence. In medical scenario this implies treatment should be allotted by clinician in the best interest of patients. Here treatment should be allotted in best patient interest rather than doctors himself. Very unfortunately patient beneficence is not regularly follows in our clinical practice. Cut practice from specialty doctors known for referral services, cut from laboratories for investigations resulting practices of unnecessary list of investigations and cut from medical store resulting in prescription of unnecessary costly medicines.
- **Dignity and honesty of doctor**
- **Avoid undue patient advantage**

Patient's Rights

The fundamental rights which describe the specific standards, principles or norms of human behavior and are regularly protected as legal rights, irrespective of nation, location, religion or any other status are known as human rights. These rights are applicable for everyone irrespective of individual. If these are applicable to all of us, it is our duty to obey their regulations and always act everyday to prevent or damages rights of others. Nowadays worldwide human rights became one strong movement. Constitution of India provides for fundamental rights, which include freedom of religion, freedom of speech, freedom of movement within the country and abroad etc. According to MCI, the doctor should not torture or act in any means that may lead to violation of human rights. Along with human rights the doctors should be aware regarding patient's rights as ethical and social responsibility.

- Right to best quality medical care and treatment
- Freedom and choice for treatment (autonomy)
- Right of self determination
- Right to religious faith and comprehension
- Right to information
- Patient confidentiality
- Informed consent

PATIENT COMMUNICATION ABILITIES

While considering communication abilities with patient, the doctors should adopt following simple principles in his mind and approach.

- He should be respectful towards his patients. Even sometimes there are some situations in which doctors are in such context so that he could not attend the patient properly. This is routinely happens in government hospitals where he is expecting heavy rush daily.
- However, even such situations, the doctor's temper should be cool and calm and he should assist the patient.
- Empathic manner during patient treatment course especially in emergency care management.

• The doctor's ethical approach plays a vital role in reflecting his good communication skills. By considering autonomy as a basic parameter for healthcare, the medical and ethical perspective both benefit from the implied reference to health.

In applying and advancing scientific knowledge, medical practice and associated technologies, human vulnerability should be taken into account. Individuals and groups of special vulnerability should be protected and the personal integrity of such individuals respected.

In conclusion, the **autonomy** is the right provided to the patient, simultaneously doctor's has to obey principles of **beneficence** and **non-maleficence** that means he has to provide best treatment to his patient and see his patient should not suffer from any harm during the treatment. The base of medical ethics stands on this conclusion which extends with provision of **justice**. Patient justice is the first duty of any doctor.

Tom Beauchamp and James Childress framed their model of medical bioethics on this concept and proposed these four parameters as **basic fundamental principles of medical bioethics**.

CONCLUSION

1. Effective communication is always consider good health indicator of concerned doctor in community.
2. Our knowledge may not change our attitude but our experience will definitely change our attitude.
3. Every communication has a content and relationship aspect.
4. Always be a good listener.
5. The doctor's caring and sharing approach plays a vital role in communication.
6. Medical confidentiality is an important extended principle of medical bioethics along with informed consent.

29

Bioethics Education in Preclinical Medical Curriculum

[The Pond report, Need of medical ethics in preclinical years, Strengths and weaknesses of ethics teaching, Course Content, Assessment Pattern, Faculty Resources, Obstacles to Ethics Education]

Background

Nowadays medical ethics education has become a universal component of undergraduate formal medical training in most countries. From the standpoint of vertical integration, medical ethics should be taught step by step throughout preclinical and clinical education. However, examples of well-integrated ethics programmers, quite often found in the literature, are mostly limited to Western industrialized countries.[1] Significant progress has been made in developing the place of ethics in undergraduate medical curricula over the last two decades.[2]

The increase in bioethics education in preclinical curricula trains and aware medical students to recognize ethical issues and determine right action.[3] Formal teaching of ethics in the medical school curriculum has increased greatly during the past 15 years. Yet, there is noted variations in their teaching pattern, syllabus framework, assessment tools, etc.[4] In India, Medical Council of India (MCI) has proposed bioethics as compulsory part of curriculum in preclinical years of students since current academic year. Present review article underlines the importance of training of bioethics and challenges in implementation in preclinical medical curricula.

The Pond Report

This movement of bioethics implementation in medical curricula really started with the Pond Report, which considered the area of ethics in medical education and made recommendations for the development of ethics teaching.[5] Subsequently, the General Medical Council's (GMC) report on undergraduate medical education, doctors, recommended the inclusion of "ethics and legal issues relevant to the practice of medicine" as a knowledge objective and "an awareness of the moral and ethical responsibilities involved in individual patient care and in the provision of care to populations of patients" as an attitudinal objective.[6] By 1997, most medical schools had a written syllabus and provided summative assessment in ethics, but there was still an urgent need for full time teachers.[7]

Need of Medical Ethics in Preclinical Years

When medical students enter in the the final year, they abruptly face complex relationship with patients, family members, consultants, residents, nurses, and with each another as professionals. These relationships may immerse students in ethically charged situations. Formal teaching of ethics in the medical school curriculum has increased greatly during the past 15 years.

Medical ethics education is instruction that endeavors to teach the examination of the role of values in the doctor's relationship with patients, colleagues, and society. It is one front of a broad curricular effort to develop physicians' values, social perspectives, and interpersonal skills for the practice of medicine.

Medical ethics training is not based on traditional teaching pattern, henceforth found difficult to implement. The urge behind such training is mainly advances in technologies and consequent horizons developed by them and lacking in ethical practices in clinic. Knowledge-based teaching found smaller area than developing cognitive skills necessary for ethical decision making. Students' exposure to media and internet has changed their personal development. Student's personal values, attitudes and behaviors is also linked with training in medical ethics.[2]

Strengths and Weaknesses of Ethics Teaching

Well-integrated syllabus pattern, small group teaching, special examination-oriented study modules, clinical teachers involvement, training, opportunities for peer analysis/ assessment, and timeliness of the teaching provide strength to ethics teaching in medical universities.

Weakness identified by many authors that need for greater integration framework, heavy theoretical concepts of ethics, literature language, lack of time, lack of resources, lack of workshops and staff developmental activities, regular knowledge brushing, ensuring practical learning, core of learning with regular learning are noted major reasons which are factors that unpopular medical ethics in medical curricula.[2] Small group teaching is widely accepted to be the best approach for classroom based teaching in this survey, although respondents observed that certain topics could be covered adequately by a didactic delivery.[2]

Course Content

After search and recent review, it was found that there is observed variations in the content of ethics curricula across the world. This reflects an emerging awareness among students, teachers and policymakers. As students are under developing stage, they may see different concepts of ethical dilemma. Genetic counseling is most challenging and difficult to accept by patients. Hence this topic is included by majority of the institutions. Secondly, the commercial support is increasing nowadays for basic research in medical institutions and their importance is increased. Hence professionalism, financial incentive ethics and conflict of interest are also included by majority of universities. Obviously inclusion of basic concepts in medical ethics like autonomy, privacy, beneficence, euthanasia, medical confidentiality, etc. are included in preclinical ethics curricula. As students of anatomy embalming, body decomposition, organ donation etc topics are included in preclinical ethics syllabus. Animal ethics is also finds topic of interest by many physiology departments from worldwide universities. As paraclinical curricula profes-sionalism, research ethics, conflict of interest, drug related ethical issues are included. However, very few medical institutions chose humanities topic area in bioethics curricula.[8,9]

Assessment Pattern

The pattern of assessment also finds challenging in medical ethics education. In United States and Canada, compulsory theoretical–practical based examination pattern is formed. Equal weightage is devoted to medical ethics, henceforth student's starts studying hard and theory pattern increase seeding act while practical approach increases their psychomotor skills with change in attitude.[10]

A recent report by the Association of American Medical Colleges (AAMC) argues that medical schools "must ensure that before graduation a student will have demonstrated . . . knowledge of the theories and principles that govern ethical decision making and of the major ethical dilemmas in medicine".[8]

Faculty Resources

There is noticed faculty pattern of variations. In some schools part time faculties are recruited from other other working departments from same universities. While in some schools full time trained faculties are appointed. Some institutions formed core group or bioethics cell with active supporting student's wings. These bioethics core team regularly conduct classes in specified timeframe like two classes per week, etc. Bioethics cell also promotes faculties' updates workshops and sharing knowledge based concepts increases their curiosity and increment in knowledge.

As medical bioethics curriculum mainly focuses preclinical departments, hence widely faculties are chosen from these departments. Secondly, students are more linked to these faculties in their early years.

The principal medical ethics course faculties tended to hold degree from clinical area although these are working in preclinical departments. In one survey study conducted over large sample size, Friedman et al noted, most deans (70%) reported there was a faculty member at their school whose primary responsibility was to teach medical ethics to medical students. Although full-time ethics researchers were less common (56%).[11]

Institutional Structure for Ethics Education[12,13]

In many institutions separate core department is formed including faculties from preclinical and clinical settings. These core departments independently handles routine curriculum activities as well as assessment. Very few universities found with specialized trained doctors as part of cell or department.

Obstacles to Ethics Education [13–15]

There is noticed number of obstacles in implementation of medical ethics in curriculum of many medical universities across the world.

Lack of time: Due to heavy schedule and exposure to new terminologies of medical field finds lack of time to both students and medical faculties to grasp these concepts of medical ethics.

Resistance from faculties: Faculty resistance is another big noted obstacle.

Limited availability of trained faculties: This is also big lacuna observed in various reviews over this aspect. This is noticeably seen due to limited training resources especially in Asian countries. However, it is a ray of hope that after compulsion by Medical Council of India, many bioethics cells are activated within very short span of time. Many major universities from India, like Maharashtra University of Health sciences, Nasik, SRM University, Manipal University, Gujarat university, etc. seriously started their training workshops over broader range.

Limited availability of literature and textbooks: This is also a major issue. Majority literature and textbooks are written from experts from the USA, Canada and other established countries. These authors framed these books according to their needs from that culture and society and literature format language is another big issue.

Specialized syllabus terminology: This is one of great challenges to faculties to teach these theoretical based concepts and along with improvement in psychomotor skills of ethics.

Interdisciplinary coordination: During working in bioethics cell, interdisciplinary coordination will be the major challenge. Medical ethics is implemented by various developed countries before 2002. However, Medical Council of India (MCI) has proposed bioethics as compulsory part of curriculum in preclinical years of students since current academic year. This will definitely change the scenario of medical ethics education in preclinical years. As assessment is going as part of university examination, the students view will be more serious. This will definitely found fruitful in future of medical education and clinical practice in India.

This chapter was published as review article in *International Journal of Healthcare and Biomedical Research*, July 2015, 3(4): 8–12 [www.ijhbr.com]

Reprinted for this textbook with prior official permission from editorial board of journal and is written by Dr MC Tayade, the same author of this textbook.

References

1. Fulford K W, Yates A, Hope T. Ethics and the GMC core curriculum: a survey of resources in UK medical schools. J Med Ethics 19972382–87.87 [PMC free article] [PubMed]

2. K Mattick and J Bligh, Teaching and assessing medical ethics: where are we now?, J Med Ethics. 2006 Mar; 32(3): 181–185.

3. Kelly E, Nisker J., Increasing bioethics education in preclinical medical curricula: what ethical dilemmas do clinical clerks experience? Acad Med. 2009 Apr;84(4):498–504. doi: 10.1097/ACM.0b013e31819a8b30.

4. Charles M. Culver, D., K. Danner Clouser, Bernard Gert, Howard Brody, John Fletcher et al, Basic Curricular Goals in Medical Ethics, N Engl J Med 1985; 312:253–256, January 24, 1985, DOI: 10.1056/NEJM198501243120430

5. Institute of Medical Ethics The Pond report: report of a working party on the teaching of medical ethics. London: IME Publications, 1987.

6. General Medical Council Tomorrow's doctors: recommendations on undergraduate medical education. p. 1993.

7. Fulford K W, Yates A, Hope T. Ethics and the GMC core curriculum: a survey of resources in UK medical schools. J Med Ethics 19972382–87.87 [PMC free article] [PubMed]

8. Jacobson JA, Tolle SW, Stocking C, Siegler M. Internal medicine residents' preferences regarding medical ethics education. Acad Med. 1989;64:760–4.

9. Martin JB, Kasper DL. In whose best interest? Breaching the academic-industrial wall, N Engl J Med. 2000;343:1646–9.

10. Christakis DA, Freudtner MA. Ethics in a short white coat: the ethical dilemmas that medical students confront. Acad Med. 1993; 68:249–54.

11. Friedman LD. The precarious position of the medical humanities in the medical school curriculum. Acad Med. 2002;77:320–2.

12. Fox E, Arnold RM, Brody B. Medical ethics education: past, present, future. Acad Med. 1995;70:761–9

13. Silverberg L I. Survey of medical ethics in US medical schools: a descriptive study. J Am Osteopath Assoc 2000100373–378.378 [PubMed]

14. Self D J, Wolinsky F D, Baldwin D C. The effect of teaching medical ethics on medical students' moral reasoning. Acad Med 198964755–759.759 [PubMed]

15. Goldie J, Schwartz L, McConnachie A. *et al.* Impact of a new course on students' potential behaviour on encountering ethical dilemmas. Med Educ 200135295–302.302 [PubMed]

Bibliography

"1120-Individual Objectivity". Institute of Internal Auditors. Retrieved July 7, 2011.

"1915 San Francisco Panama-Pacific International Exposition: In color!". National Museum American History. February 11, 2011. Retrieved July 14, 2011.

"1Mb Broadband Access Becomes Legal Right". YLE (Helsinki). October 14, 2009. Retrieved December 15, 2011.

"A Single-Issue Political Party for Longevity Science". Fight Aging!. Retrieved 20 April 2015.

Abrams, J.L. Embalming. 2008.

Adam Schroeder. In the Fabled East: A Novel. D and M Publishers. p. 174.

Ader, Petkas, and Blackwell, Whistleblowing (1972).

Adler, Mortimer J., ed. et al. (1952). The Great Ideas: A Syntopicon of Great Books of the Western World. Chicago: Encyclopædia Britannica. p. 788.

"African Commission on Human and Peoples' Rights". Achpr.org. July 20, 1979. Retrieved August 29, 2010.

"Aging and Death in an Organism That Reproduces by Morphologically Symmetric Division" (PDF).

AIAA (2007). "Publication Ethical Standards: Guidelines and Procedures". AIAA Jl 45 (8): 1794. doi:10.2514/1.32639.

Alain Pellet "Droits-de-l'hommisme" et droit international 2000.

Alleyne, Richard (November 20, 2008). "Scientists take a step closer to an elixir of youth". The Daily Telegraph (London). Retrieved May 5, 2010.

American Psychological Association. (2002). "2010 Amendments to the American Psychological Association ethical principles of psychologists and code of conduct.".

"Americans want to water down Helsinki Declaration". Bulletin of medical ethics 136: 3–4. 1998. PMID 11657531.

Amnesty International Report 2005 Report 2006 at the Wayback Machine (archived March 17, 2007)

Anderman, Gunilla M.; Rogers, Margaret (2003). Translation Today: Trends and Perspectives. Multilingual Matters. Retrieved 1 January 2012.

Angell M (October 1988). "Ethical imperialism? Ethics in international collaborative clinical research". The New England Journal of Medicine 319 (16): 1081–3.doi:10.1056/NEJM 198810203191608. PMID 3173435.

Anger, Margaret (1920). Woman and the New Race. Brentano. p. 100.

Annas, Glantz, Katz, George, Leonard, Barbara (1977). Informed Consent to Human Experimentation. Cambridge, Massa-chusetts: Ballinger Publishing Company. pp. 63–93. ISBN 0-88410-147-9.

"Anthropologists have moral obligations as members of other groups, such as the family, religion, and community, as well as the profession. They also have obligations to the scholarly discipline, to the wider society and culture, and to the human species, other species, and the environment"

Appel, JM. Must My Doctor Tell My Partner? Rethinking Confidentiality In the HIV Era, Medicine and Health Rhode Island, Jun 2006.

Article 20(1). European Convention on Human Rights and Biomedicine (1997). Adopted at Oviedo, 4 April 1997.

Attorney-General v Observer Ltd [1990] 1 A.C. 109

Autonomy in Moral and Political Philosophy (Stanford Encyclopedia of Philosophy). Plato.stanford.edu. Retrieved on 2013-07-12.

Babbie, Earl (2010). The practice of social research (12th ed.). Belmont, Calif: Wadsworth Cengage. ISBN 0495598410.

"Bacteria Death Reduces Human Hopes of Immortality". New Scientist magazine, issue 2485, page 19. February 5, 2005. Retrieved 2007-04-02.

Baker, Nena (2008). The Body Toxic. North Point Press. p. 142. cited from Lessig 2011, p. 25.

Ball, Olivia; Gready, Paul (2006). The no-nonsense guide to human rights. New Internationalist (Oxford). ISBN 978-1-904456-45-2.

Baumrind, D. (1964). "Some thoughts on ethics of research: After reading Milgram's "Behavioral Study of Obedience."". American Psychologist 19 (6): 421.doi:10.1037/h0040128. edit

Baumslag, Naomi (2005). Murderous Medicine: Nazi Doctors, Human Experimentation, and Typhus. Praeger Publishers. pp. xxv. ISBN 9780275983123.

Bayles, Michael; Bruce Chapman (1983). Ethical Issues in the Law of Tort. New York: Springer-Verlag. pp. 20–21. ISBN 90-277-1639-0.

Beauchamp, Tom L.; Childress, James F. (1994). Principles of Biomedical Ethics (Fourth ed.). New York: Oxford University Press. ISBN 0-19-508536-1.

Beauchamp, Tom L.; Davidson, Arnold I. (1979). "The Definition of Euthanasia". Journal of Medicine and Philosophy 4 (3): 294–312. doi:10.1093/jmp/4.3.294.PMID 501249.

Beitz, Charles R. (2009). The idea of human rights. Oxford: Oxford University Press. ISBN 978-0-19-957245-8.

Bekelman JE, Li Y, Gross CP (2003), "Scope and impact of financial conflicts of interest in biomedical research: a systematic review". JAMA 289 (4): 454–65.doi:10.1001/jama.289.4.454. PMID 12533125.

Belinda Cooper (book reviewer), September 24, 2010, The New York Times, New Birth of Freedom, Retrieved Aug. 14, 2014

Berlant, Jeffrey, Profession and Monopoly: a study of medicine in the United States and Great Britain. University of California Press, 1975, ISBN 0-520-02734-5.

Bernstein C, Bernstein H. (1991) Aging, Sex, and DNA Repair. Academic Press, San Diego. ISBN 0120928604 ISBN 978-0120928606

"Bill to amend RTI Act deferred to Winter Session". thehindubusinessline.com. Retrieved 13 September 2013.

"Biocentrism". Encyclopædia Britannica. 2009. Retrieved 13 March 2009.

"Bioethics Society of Cornell". Cornell University. Archived from the original on 17 June 2012.

Blake R, Early E (1995). "Patients' attitudes about gifts to physicians from pharmaceutical companies". J Am Board Fam Pract 8 (6): 457–64. PMID 8585404.

Bloustein, Edward J. (1964). "Privacy as an Aspect of Human Dignity: An Answer to Dean Prosser". New York University Law Review (962): 973–974.

Bok, Sissela (1989). Secrets : on the ethics of concealment and revelation (Vintage Books ed. ed.). New York: Vintage Books. pp. 10–11. ISBN 978-0679724735.

Borry P, Schotsmans P, Dierickx K (April 2006). "Empirical research in bioethical journals. A quantitative analysis". J Med Ethics 32 (4): 240–5. doi:10.1136/jme.2004.011478.PMC 2565792. PMID 16574880.

Bourdieu, 2001 (MARANHÃO, 2005; 2006; 2007; SOBRAL and MARANHÃO, 2008.

Boyd, Danah. "What does the Facebook experiment teach us?". Social Media Collective Research Blog. Retrieved April 26, 2015.

Brennan TA (August 1999). "Proposed revisions to the Declaration of Helsinki—will they weaken the ethical principles underlying human research?". The New England Journal of Medicine 341 (7): 527–31. doi:10.1056/NEJM199908123410712. PMID 10441612.

Bruce E. Johansen (September 1998). "Sterilization of Native American Women". Native Americas.

Bruckman A (2002). "Studying the amateur artist: A perspective on disguising data collected in human subjects research on the Internet". Ethics and Information Technology 4 (3): 217–31. oi:10.1023/A:1021316409277.

Burns H. Weston, March 20, 2014, Encyclopedia Britannica, human rights, Retrieved Aug. 14, 2014.

Burns, Chester R. (1977). Legacies in ethics and medicine. New York: Science History Publications. ISBN 9780882021669. In this book see Mary Catherine Welborn's excerpts from her 1966 The long tradition: A study in fourteenth-century medical deontology.

Burns, Chester R. (1977). Legacies in ethics and medicine. New York: Science History Publications. ISBN 9780882021669. In this book see De Mondeville's "On the morals and ethics of medicine" from Ethics in Medicine.

Cameron, M. E. "Book Reviews." The American Journal of Nursing 13.1 (1912):75-77. JSTOR. Web. 10 April 2010. [2]

Campbell v MGN Ltd [2004] 2 A.C. 457

Carlson, Robert V.; Boyd, Kenneth M.; Webb, David J. (2004). "The revision of the Declaration of Helsinki: past, present and future". British Journal of Clinical Pharmacology 57 (6): 695–713. doi:10.1111/j.1365-2125.2004.02103.x.PMC 1884510. PMID 15151515.

Carney, Scott. "The Case for Mandatory Organ Donation". Wired. Conde Naste. Retrieved 13 February 2015.

Carole Ruth McCann. Birth control politics in the United States, 1916–1945. Cornell University Press. p. 100.

Castagnera, James (Spring 2003). "The Rise of the Whistleblower and the Death of Privacy Impact of 9/11 and Enron". Labor Law Journal.

Center for Drug Evaluation and Research. Guidance for industry: acceptance of foreign clinical studies. March, 2001.

Chalil Madathil, K.; Koikkara, R.; Obeid, J.; Greenstein, J. S.; Sanderson, I. C.; Fryar, K.; Moskowitz, J.; Gramopadhye, A. K. (2013). "An investigation of the efficacy of electronic consenting interfaces of research permissions management system in a hospital setting". International Journal of Medical Informatics 82 (9): 854–863.doi:10.1016/j.ijmedinf.2013.04.008. PMC 3779682. PMID 23757370.

Chapple, Christopher. "Hinduism, Jainism, and Ecology". Patheos.com. Retrieved 3 December 2012.

Chapter 17, 'Letting People Choose for Themselves', of 'How to Make Good Decisions and Be Right All the Time', Iain King, Continuum, 2008, ISBN 978-1847-063-472.

"Children of the Camps | Internment Timeline". Pbs.org. Retrieved August 29, 2010.

Christie B (October 2000). "Doctors revise Declaration of Helsinki". BMJ 321 (7266): 913. doi:10.1136/bmj.321.7266.913. PMC 1118720. PMID 11030663.

Clark, W.R. 1999. A Means to an End: The biological basis of aging and death. New York: Oxford University Press. [1] About telomeres and programmed cell death.

"Classification of diseases functioning and disability".

Coco v A N Clark (Engineers) Ltd; ChD 1969.

Codes of Ethics, Some History, Center for the Study of Ethics in the Professions at IIT, Downloaded on 12.11.2014

Committee on Bioethics. Informed consent, parental permission, and assent in pediatric practice. Pediatrics 1995;95(2):314–7.

"Compound resveratrol may turn off a protein that guards cancer cells from cancer-fighting therapies". Wordpress. rudramani. com. 2009-07-13. Retrieved 2010-11-04.

Copland, James (1 March 1825). "The Hippocratic Oath". The London Medical Repository 23 (135): 258. Retrieved 22 September 2014.. For the Greek text, see Jones, W. H. S., ed. (1868). Hippocrates Collected Works (in Greek) I. Cambridge Harvard University Press. pp. 130–131. Retrieved 22 September 2014.

Corp Ltd v First Netcom Pty Ltd (1997) 148 ALR 202 at 208.

"Corporations and Human Rights". Human Rights Watch. Archived from the originalon December 15, 2007.

Council for International Organization of Medical Sciences (CIOMS) and World Health Organization (WHO) Geneva, Switzerland, 2002.

"International Ethical Guidelines for Biomedical Research Involving Human Subjects" (PDF).

Council for International Organizations of Medical Sciences (1993). "Guideline 11: Selection of pregnant or nursing (breast-feeding) women as research subjects". International Ethical Guidelines for Biomedical Research Involving Human Subjects. Geneva: World Health Organisation. ISBN 92-9036-056-9.

Creel, Herrlee G. (1982). What is Taoism? : and other studies in Chinese cultural history. Chicago: University of Chicago Press. p. 17. ISBN 0226120473.

Critchlow, Donald T. (1999). Intended Consequences: Birth Control, Abortion, and the Federal Government in Modern America. New York: Oxford University Press. p. 15.

Curry, Patrick (2006). Ecological ethics: an introduction. Polity. p. 60. ISBN 978-0-7456-2908-7.

Custodial deaths in West Bengal and India's refusal to ratify the Convention against Torture Asian Human Rights Commission 26 February 2004.

D. Mavinic (2006). "The "Art" of Plagiarism". Canadian Journal of Civil Engineering 33 (3): iii–vi.

Dag Øistein Endsjø. Greek Resurrection Beliefs and the Success of Christianity. New York: Palgrave Macmillan 2009; cf. Dag Øistein Endsjø "Immortal Bodies, Before Christ. Bodily Continuity in Ancient Greece and 1 Corinthians" in Journal for the Study of the New Testament 30 (2008):417–36.

Darwin, Charles. "Notebook B: [Transmutation of species]". Retrieved 30 October 2012.

de Grey, Aubrey; Rae, Michael (September 2007). Ending Aging: The Rejuvenation Breakthroughs that Could Reverse Human Aging in Our Lifetime. New York, New York: St. Martin's Press. p. 416. ISBN 0-312-36706-6.

Dealing with—or reporting—"unacceptable" behavior (with additional thoughts about the "Bystander Effect") Mary Rowe MIT, Linda Wilcox HMS, Howard Gadlin NIH (2009), Journal of the International Ombudsman Association 2(1), online at ombudsassociation.org

Declaration of Helsinki—Current (2013) version

"Declaration on the Responsibilities of the Present Generation Towards the Future Generation". UNESCO. Retrieved August 29, 2010.

"Definitions of Genetic Testing". Definitions of Genetic Testing (Jorge Sequeiros and Bárbara Guimarães). EuroGentest Network of Excellence Project. 2008-09-11.

Delmas, Candice (January 2015). "The Ethics of Government Whisltleblowing". Social Theory and Practice.

Derr, Patrick George; Edward M. McNamara (2003). Case studies in environmental ethics. Rowman and Littlefield. p. 21. ISBN 978-0-7425-3137-6.

Deutsch E, Taupitz J. Göttingen Report. Freedom and control of biomedical research- the planned revision of the Declaration of Helsinki. Wld Med J 1999 45: 40-41

Doebbler, Curtis F. J (2006). Introduction to international human rights law. Cd Publishing. ISBN 978-0-9743570-2-7.

Dolan, SM (Aug 2009). "Prenatal genetic testing". Pediatric annals 38 (8): 426–30.doi:10.3928/00904481-20090723-05. PMID 19711880.

Donnelly, Jack (2003). Universal human rights in theory and practice (2nd ed.). Ithaca: Cornell University Press. ISBN 978-0-8014-8776-7.

Dorr G, Logan A. Quality, not mere quantity counts: black eugenics and the NAACP baby contests. In: Lombardo P, ed. A Century of Eugenics in America. Bloomington, Ind.: Indiana University Press; 2011:68–92.

Dorr, Gregory (2008). Segregation's Science. Charlottesville: University of Virginia Press. p. 10.

Dorr, Gregory Michael. "Encyclopedia Virginia: Buck v Bell". Retrieved May 3, 2011.

Dr Coburn's Peculiar Privilege, 2 October 2009

Dr Motilal C Tayade, Dr Vinod, Dr Ramchandra G Latti, Translational research in physiology: Review, Indian Journal of Basic and Applied Medical Research; June 2015: Vol. 4, Issue 3, P. 405–414.

Dr Motilal C. Tayade, Dr Sunil M. Bhamare, Dr Prathamesh Kamble, Dr. Kirankumar Jadhav, Review: Writing good research paper: Advice for beginners, Indian Journal of Basic and Applied Medical Research; March 2013: 6(2), P. 460–463.

Dr Prathamesh Kamble, Dr Motilal Tayade, Dr Shital Maske, Dr Kirankumar Jadhav, Dr Sunil Bhamare, Editorial Review: Encyclopedia of DNA Elements (ENCODE) Project: A Major Scientific Milestone, International J. of Healthcare and Biomedical Research, Volume: 1, Issue: 1, October 2012 P: 1–5

Draper, Heather (1998). "Euthanasia". In Chadwick, Ruth. Encyclopedia of Applied Ethics 2. Academic Press.

Duncan, Francesca E; Jozefik, Jennifer K; Kim, Alison M; Hirshfeld-Cytron, Jennifer; Woodruff, Teresa K (2011). "The Gynecologist Has a Unique Role in Providing Oncofertility Care to Young Cancer Patients". US Obstetrics and Gynaecology 6 (1): 24–34. PMC 3171692. PMID 21927621.

Durham, H. (2004). ""We the People: The Position of NGOs in Gathering Evidence and Giving Witness in International Criminal Trials". In Thakur, R, Malcontent, P. From Sovereign Impunity to International Accountability. New York: United Nations University Press.

Edelstein, Jason (October 12, 2010). "The Search for the Truth". The Jerusalem Post.

Edelstein, Ludwig (1943). The Hippocratic Oath: Text, Translation and Interpretation. p. 56. ISBN 978-0-8018-0184-6.

Ellis, Karen and Jodie Keane (November 2008). "Do we need a new 'Good for Development' label?". Overseas Development Institute.

Elof Axel Carlson (2001). The unfit: a history of a bad idea. p. 193.ISBN 9780879695873. Retrieved July 14, 2011.

Eltier, James W., Anthony M. Allessandro, and Andrew J. Dahl. "Use of Social Media and College Student Organizations to Increase Support for Organ Donation and Advocacy: A Case Report." Progress in Transplantation (2012): 436–41. EBSCO. Web. 29 June 2014.

Entlicher, D. (January 01, 2009). Presumed consent to organ donation: its rise and fall in the united STATES. Rutgers Law Review, 61, 2, 295.

Mortimer Adler et al. (1952). The Great Ideas: A Syntopicon of Great Books of the Western World. Chicago: Encyclopædia Britannica. p. 784.

Euthanasia and assisted suicide BBC. Last reviewed June 2011. Accessed 25 July 2011. Archived from the original here. The Dutch law however, does not use the term 'euthanasia' but includes it under the broader definition of "assisted suicide and termination of life on request."See:http://www.schreeu-womleven.nl/abortus/text_of_dutch_euthanasia_law.doc. See also:Euthanasia in the Netherlands.

Euthanasia and Law in the Netherlands—Page 186, John Griffiths, Alex Bood, Heleen Weyers—1998

Eysenbach G, Till JE (2001). "Ethical issues in qualitative research on internet communities". BMJ 323 (7321): 1103–5. doi:10.1136/bmj.323.7321.1103.PMC 59687. PMID 11701577.

Faden, R. R.; Beauchamp, T. L. (1986). A History and Theory of Informed Consent. New York: Oxford University Press. ISBN 0-19-503686-7.

Faunce, T.A. "Developing and Teaching the Virtue-Ethics Foundations of Healthcare Whistle Blowing", Monash Bioethics Review. 2004; 23(4): 41–55.

Fernandez, Soraya (December 9, 2008). "Protecting access to markets". COPLA. Archived from the original on April 29, 2011.

"FindLaw's Writ-Amar: Executive Privilege". Writ.corporate. findlaw.com. 2004-04-16. Retrieved 2012-01-01.

"First nation makes broadband access a legal right". CNN. July 12, 2010. Retrieved December 15, 2011.

"Fixing the Fourth Amendment with trade secret law: A response to Kyllo v. United States". Georgetown Law Journal. 2002.

"Four in Five Regard Internet Access as a Fundamental Right: Global Poll" (PDF). BBC News. Retrieved December 15, 2011.

Francis Bacon: The Major Works by Francis Bacon, edited by Brian Vickers, p. 630.

Fred Grünfeld and Anke Huijboom, The failure to prevent genocide in Rwanda: the role of bystanders (2007), p. 199.

Frederick, L.G.; Strub, Clarence G. [1959] (1989). The Principles and Practice of Embalming, 5th ed., Dallas, TX: Professional Training Schools Inc and Robertine Frederick. OCLC 20723376.

Freeman, Michael (2002). Human rights : an interdisciplinary approach. Cambridge: Polity Press. ISBN 978-0-7456-2355-9.

Freemont, P. F.; Kitney, R. I., Synthetic Biology. New Jersey: World Scientific, 2012, ISBN 978-1-84816-862-6.

Fried, Charles (January 1968). "Privacy". Yale Law Journal 77 (3): 475–493.

Galvin, Kathleen M.; Clayman, Marla L. (2010). "Whose Future Is It? Ethical Family Decision Making About Daughters' Treatment in the Oncofertility Context". Oncofertility. Cancer Treatment and Research 156. pp. 429–45. doi:10.1007/978-1-4419-6518-9-33. ISBN 978-1-4419-6517-2. PMC 3086488. PMID 20811853.

Garrett Hardin, "The Tragedy of the Commons", Science, Vol. 162, No. 3859 (December 13, 1968), pp. 1243–1248. Also available here [4] and here.

Gartrell N, Milliken N, Goodson W, Thiemann S, Lo B (1992). "Physician-patient sexual contact. Prevalence and problems". West J Med 157 (2): 139–43. PMC 1011231.PMID 1441462.

Gavison, Ruth (1980). "Privacy and the Limits of Law". Yale Law Journal: 421–471.

General Assembly WMA Hamburg, Germany 1997.

Genetic Alliance Site [Internet]. [cited 2010 Oct 29]. Available from:http://www.geneticalliance.org/.

Gilberson, Lance, Zoology Lab Manual, 4th edition. Primis Custom Publishing. 1999.

Gilbert, Scott F. (2006). "Cheating Death: The Immortal Life Cycle of Turritopsis". Retrieved 2009-06-14.

Gillon, R (1994). "Medical ethics: four principles plus attention to scope". British Medical Journal 309 (184). doi:10.1136/bmj. 309.6948.184.

Godkin, E.L. (December 1880). "Libel and its Legal Remedy". Atlantic Monthly 46 (278): 729–739.

Goldim, J. R. (2009). Revisiting the beginning of bioethics: The contributions of Fritz Jahr (1927). Perspect Biol Med, Sum, 377–380.

Goldim, J. R., Revisiting the beginning of bioethics: The contributions of Fritz Jahr, 2009, Perspect Biol Med, Sum, 377–380.

Gordon, Linda (2003). The Moral Property of Women: A History of Birth Control Politics in America. Urbana: University of Illinois Press. p. 345. ISBN 0-252-07459-9.

Gould, Stephen J. (1981) The mismeasure of man. Norton.

Grady, Christine; Forster, Heidi P. and Emanuel, Ezekiel (October 2001). "The 2000 Revision of the Declaration of Helsinki: A Step Forward or More Confusion?". The Lancet 358 (9291): 1449–1453. doi:10.1016/S0140-6736(01)06534-5.

Gregory, John (1772). Lectures on the Duties and Qualifications of a Physician.

Grimmelmann, James. "Illegal, Immoral, and Mood-Altering How Facebook and OkCupid Broke the Law When They Experimented on Users". Medium. Retrieved April 26, 2015.

"Guideline 11: Selection of pregnant or nursing (breastfeeding) women as research subjects". International Ethical Guidelines for Biomedical Research Involving Human Subjects. Geneva: World Health Organisation. (1993) ISBN 92-9036-056-9.

Güldal D, Semin S (2000). "The influences of drug companies' advertising programs on physicians". Int J Health Serv 30 (3): 585–95. doi:10.2190/GYW9-XUMQ-M3K2-T31C.PMID 11109183.

Hamilton Cravens, The triumph of evolution: American scientists and the heredity-environment controversy, 1900–1941 (Philadelphia: University of Pennsylvania Press, 1978): 179.

Hannum, Hurst (2006). "The concept of human rights". International Human Rights: Problems of Law, Policy, And Practice. Aspen Publishers. pp. 31–33. ISBN 0735555575.

Harrison's Principles of Internal Medicine, Ch. 69, Cancer cell biology and angiogenesis, Robert G. Fenton and Dan L. Longo, p. 454.

Hayflick, L (2007). "Biological Aging is No Longer an Unsolved Problem" (PDF). Annals of the New York Academy of Sciences. doi:10.1196/annals.1395.001.

Helms, Ann Doss and Tomlinson, Tommy (26 September 2011). "Wallace Kuralt's era of sterilization: Mecklenburg's impoverished had few, if any, rights in the 1950s and 1960s as he oversaw one of the most aggressive efforts to sterilize certain populations". Charlotte Observer. Retrieved 10 December 2011.

"Health Sciences South Carolina". healthsciencessc.org. Retrieved 14 September 2014.

"Historical Background to the European Court of Human Rights". European Court of Human Rights. Archived from the original on December 22, 2007.

Hodgson, JM; Gillam, LH; Sahhar, MA; Metcalfe, SA (Feb 2010). ""Testing times, challenging choices": an Australian study of prenatal genetic counseling". Journal of genetic counseling 19 (1): 22–37. doi:10.1007/s10897-009-9248-6. PMID 19798554.

Homan, R. (1991). The Ethics of Social Research. London; New York: Longman. ISBN 0-582-05879-1.

Horrow, Aviva. "When Nature Holds the Mastery": The Development of Biocentric Thought in Industrial America". Retrieved 30 October 2012.

Hoshang, Dr. Bhadha. http://tenets.zoroastrianism.com/topi33.html

"HSSC/RPMS · GitHub". github.com. Retrieved 14 September 2014.

http://en.wikipedia.org/wiki/Bioethics Downloaded on 03/06/2015

http://en.wikipedia.org/wiki/Informed_consent Downloaded on 03/06/2015

http://icmr.nic.in/bioethics/Guidelines_medicalcollege.pdf

http://rti.gov.in/RTICorner/Guide_2013-issue.pdf

http://www.aftenposten.no/nyheter/iriks/22juli/Tingretten-ber-Behring-Breiviks-mor-om-unnskyldning-6912500.html

http://www.mciindia.org/RulesandRegulations/Code of Medical Ethics Regulations2002.aspx

http://www.ncsl.org/IssuesResearch/Health/AbortionLaws/tabid/14401/Default.aspx#parent

http://www.nsgc.org/About/FAQsDefinitions/tabid/97/Default.aspx

http://www.nsgc.org/About/FAQsDefinitions/tabid/97/Default.aspx

http://www.ohchr.org/EN/Issues/Pages/What are Human Rights.aspx Downloaded on 06/07/2015

http://www.unfpa.org/human-rights

Hubert Chanson (2007). "Research Quality, Publications and Impact in Civil Engineering into the 21st Century. Publish or Perish, Commercial versus Open Access, Internet versus Libraries ?". Canadian Journal of Civil Engineering 34 (8): 946–951. doi:10.1169/L07-027.

Hubert Chanson (2008). Digital Publishing, Ethics and Hydraulic Engineering: The Elusive or "Boring" Bore?. In: Stefano Pagliara 2nd International Junior Researcher and Engineer Workshop on Hydraulic Structures (IJREW'08), Pisa, Italy, Keynote, pp. 3–13, 30 July–1 August 2008. ISBN 978-88-8492-568-8.

Human D, Fluss S. The World Medical Association's Declaration of Helsinki: Historical and contemporary perspectives. 5th draft. WMA 2001

"Human rights: A crowded field". The Economist (London). May 27, 2010. Retrieved August 9, 2010.

"Human Rights: Statement on Human Rights, Sexual Orientation and Gender Identity at High Level Meeting". Mission of the Netherlands to the UN. June 3, 2008. Retrieved August 29, 2010.

Human Rights in the Twentieth Century, edited by Stefan-Ludwig Hoffmann, Introduction: Genealogies of Human Rights, Retrieved Aug. 14, 2014.

Iconi T. Evolution and complexity: the double-edged sword. Artif Life. 2008 14(3–325–44)

"Immortal' jellyfish swarming across the world". London: Telegraph Media Group. January 30, 2009. Retrieved 2009-06-14.

"Immortality: definition of immortality in Oxford dictionary (American English) (US)". Retrieved 20 April 2015.

"India: Repeal the Armed Forces Special Powers Act, Law Provides Impunity for Human Rights Abuses, Fuels Cycles of Violence", Human Rights Watch, 21 November 2007

"India: The Jammu and Kashmir Public Safety Act—a threat to human rights", AI Index ASA 20/019/2000, Amnesty Inter-national, 15 May 2000

Indiana Supreme Court Legal History Lecture Series, "Three Generations of Imbeciles are Enough:"Reflections on 100 Years of Eugenics in Indiana, at In.gov

Information Privacy, Official Reference for the Certified Information privacy Professional (CIPP), Swire, P. P. [1]. and Bermann, S. (2007).

Ingram, David; Jennifer Parks (2002). The complete idiot's guide to understanding ethics. Alpha Books. p. 201. ISBN 978-0-02-864325-0.

"Internet access is 'a fundamental right'". BBC News. March 8, 2010. Retrieved December 15, 2011.

J. Mitchell Miller (2009-08-06). 21st Century Criminology: A Reference Handbook, Volume 1. p. 193. ISBN 9781412960199. Retrieved July 15, 2011.

Jackson, John P. and Weidman, Nadine M. (2005). Race, racism, and science: social impact and interaction. Rutgers University Press. p. 123. ISBN 978-0-8135-3736-8.

James Nickel, with assistance from Thomas Pogge, M.B.E. Smith, and Leif Wenar, Dec 13, 2013, Stanford Encyclopedia of Philosophy, Human Rights.

"Jammu and Kashmir Public Safety Act, 1978 (Act No. 6 of 1978)", Refworld, High Commissioner for Refugees, United Nations

Jeffay, Nathan (June 24, 2010). "Academic hits out at politicised charities". The Jewish Chronicle.

JH Medicine Policy on Interaction with Industry effective date July 1, 2009, accessed July 20, 2011.

JM Appel. May Physicians Date Their Patients' Relatives? Rethinking Sexual Misconduct and Disclosure After Long v. Ostroff, Medicine and Health, Rhode Island, May 2004.

Joel Garreau (October 31, 2007). "The Invincible Man". The Washington Post: C01.

Johnson, Jayme. "Biocentric Ethics and the Inherent Value of Life" (PDF). umass.edu. Retrieved 10 November 2012.

Jones, Nicola and Hayley Baker (March 2008). "Untangling links between trade, poverty and gender". Overseas Development Institute.

Jordan, M. C. (1998). "Ethics manual. Fourth edition. American College of Physicians".Ann Intern Med 128 (7): 576–94. doi:10.1001/archinte.128.4.576. PMID 9518406.

J. Shyamantha, Asokan (11 December 2013). "India's Supreme Court turns the clock back with gay sex ban". Reuters.

Judi Bari (1995). "Revolutionary Ecology: Biocentrism and Deep Ecology". Alarm: A Journal of Revolutionary Ecology.

Jungheim, Emily S.; Carson, Kenneth R.; Brown, Douglas (2010). "Counseling and Consenting Women with Cancer on Their Oncofertility Options: A Clinical Perspective". Oncofertility. Cancer Treatment and Research 156. pp. 403–12. doi:10.1007/978-1-4419-6518-9_31. ISBN 978-1-4419-6517-2. PMC 3071538. PMID 20811851.

Karandikar PM,Tayade MC, Application of Robotics technology in clinical practice in India, Asian Journal of Medical Sciences, September 2013, Vol. 5(1), 29–33.

Katz, Jay; Alexander Morgan Capron (2002). The silent world of doctor and patient(Johns Hopkins Paperbacks ed.). Baltimore: Johns Hopkins University Press. pp. 7–9.ISBN 978-0801857805.

Kaur, Jaskaran (2004). Twenty Years of Impunity: The November 1984 Pogroms of Sikhs in India.

Kerr, Robert S. "Senator Kerr Talks about Conflict of Interest", U.S. News and World Report, September 3, 1962, p. 86.

Kimmelman, J.; Weijer, C; Meslin, E (2009). "Helsinki discords: FDA, ethics, and international drug trials". The Lancet 373 (9657): 13–4. doi:10.1016/S0140-6736(08)61936-4. PMID 19121708.

Kirkwood, T.B.L. 1977. Evolution of aging. Nature, 270: 301–304. [3] Origin of the disposable soma theory.

Kline, Wendy (2005). Building a Better Race: Gender, Sexuality, and Eugenics From the Turn of the Century to the Baby Boom. University of California Press. p. 4.

Kluchin, Rebecca M. (2009). Fit to Be Tied: Sterilization and Reproductive Rights in America 1950–1980. New Brunswick: Rutgers University Press. pp. 17–20.

Kohl, Marvin (1974). The Morality of Killing. New York: Humanities Press. p. 94., quoted in Beauchamp and Davidson (1979), p 294. A similar definition is offered by Blackburn (1994) with "the action of causing the quick and painless death of a person, or not acting to prevent it when prevention was within the agent's powers."

Kohl, Marvin; Kurtz, Paul (1975). "A Plea for Beneficient Euthanasia". In Kohl, Marvin.Beneficient Euthanasia. Buffalo, New York: Prometheus Books. p. 94., quoted in Beauchamp and Davidson (1979), p 295.

Kramer, Adam; Guillory, Jaime; Jeffrey, Hancock (2014). "Experimental evidence of massive-scale emotional contagion through social networks". PNAS 111.doi:10.1073/pnas. 1320040111.

Krauthammer, Charles. "Yes, Let's Pay for Organs". TIME. Time Inc. Retrieved 28 February 2015.

Kühl, Stefan (2002-02-14). The Nazi Connection: Eugenics, American Racism, and German National Socialism. p. 70. ISBN 9780195348781.

Kurzweil, Raymond (2005). The Singularity Is Near: When Humans Transcend Biology. Viking Adult. ISBN 0-670-03384-7.

La Puma J, Priest E (1992). "Is there a doctor in the house? An analysis of the practice of physicians' treating their own families". JAMA 267 (13): 1810–2.doi:10.1001/jama.267.13.1810. PMID 1545466.

La Puma J, Stocking C, La Voic D, Darling C (1991). "When physicians treat members of their own families. Practices in a community hospital". N Engl J Med 325 (18): 1290–4. DOI:10.1056/NEJM199110313251806. PMID 1922224.

LA Times, "Drug money withdrawals: Medical schools review rules on pharmaceutical freebies", posted 2/12/07, accessed. 3/6/07

Lakhan SE, Hamlat E, McNamee T, Laird C (2009), "Time for a unified approach to medical ethics". Philosophy, Ethics, and Humanities in Medicine 4 (3): 13.DOI:10.1186/1747-5341-4-13. PMC 2745426. PMID 19737406.

LANIER, Jaron. "Should Facebook Manipulate Users?" The New York Times. Retrieved April 26, 2015.

Larson 2004, pp. 194–195 Citing Buck v. Bell 274 U.S. 200, 205 (1927).

Larson, Edward J. (1995). Sex, Race, and Science: Eugenics in the Deep South. Baltimore: Johns Hopkins University Press. p. 75.

Lawrence, Jane (2000). "The Indian Health Service and the Sterilization of Native American Women". The American Indian Quarterly. 3 24 (3): 400–419.doi:10.1353/aiq.2000.0008.

Lee Feinstein, Darfur and beyond: what is needed to prevent mass atrocities (2007) p. 46.

"Left Biocentrism Primer". 1998-03-15. Retrieved 2009-03-15.

Lennon v News Group Newspapers Ltd (1978) FSR. 573

Leopold, Aldo (1949). Sand County Almanac. Random House Digital Inc. p. 239.

Lessig 2011, pp. 29–32

Let's (Cautiously) Celebrate the "New Eugenics", Huffington Post, (Oct. 30, 2014).

Levine RJ (August 1993). "New international ethical guidelines for research involving human subjects". Annals of Internal Medicine 119 (4): 339–41. doi:10.7326/0003-4819-119-4-199308150-00016. PMID 8328746.

Levine RJ (August 1999). "The need to revise the Declaration of Helsinki". The New England Journal of Medicine 341 (7): 531–4. doi:10.1056/NEJM199908123410713.PMID 10441613.

Levine, RJ (2000). "Some recent developments in the international guidelines on the ethics of research involving human subjects". Annals of the New York Academy of Sciences 918: 170–8. Bibcode:2000NYASA.918..170L.doi:10.1111/j.1749-6632.2000. tb05486.x. PMID 11131702.

Levitt, S. D.; List, J. A. (2007). "What Do Laboratory Experiments Measuring Social Preferences Reveal about the Real World?" Journal of Economic Perspectives 21 (2): 153–174. doi:10.1257/jep.21.2.153. JSTOR 30033722.

Levitt, S. D.; List, J. A. (2009). "Field experiments in economics: The past, the present, and the future". European Economic Review 53 (1): 1–18.doi:10.1016/j.euroecorev.2008.12.001.

Lin Kah Wai (18 April 2004). "Telomeres, Telomerase, and Tumorigenesis—A Review". MedGenMed 6 (3): 19. PMC 1435592. PMID 15520642.

List, J. A.; List, J. A. (2008). "Informed Consent in Social Science". Science 322 (5902): 672. doi:10.1126/science.322.5902.672a.

Lloyd, Geoffrey, ed. (1983). Hippocratic Writings (2nd ed.). London: Penguin Books. p. 94. ISBN 0140444513.

Lo and Field (2009). The definition originally appeared in Thompson (1993).

Loff, B; Black, J (2000). "The Declaration of Helsinki and research in vulnerable populations". The Medical journal of Australia 172 (6): 292–5. PMID 10860097.

Loff, Bebe; Gillam, Deborah; Loff, Lynn (2000). "The Declaration of Helsinki, CIOMS and the ethics of research on vulnerable populations". Nature Medicine 6 (6): 615–7.doi:10.1038/76174. PMID 10835665.

Lolas, Fernando (2008). "Bioethics and animal research: A personal perspective and a note on the contribution of Fritz Jahr". Biological Research (Santiago) 41 (1): 119–123.doi:10.4067/S0716-97602008000100013.

Lombardo, 2008: pp. 211–213.

Lombardo, 2011: p. 1.

Lombardo, 2011: p. ix.

Lombardo, Paul; "Eugenic Laws Against Race-Mixing", Eugenics Archive.

Lombardo, Paul; "Eugenic Sterilization Laws", Eugenics Archive

Lombardo, Paul; "Eugenics Laws Restricting Immigration,", Eugenics Archive.

Lucasfilm Limited v Ainsworth (2011) UKSC 39.

Lurie P, Wolfe SM; Wolfe (September 1997). "Unethical trials of interventions to reduce perinatal transmission of the human immunodeficiency virus in developing countries". The New England Journal of Medicine 337 (12): 853–6.doi:10.1056/ NEJM199709183371212. PMID 9295246.

Macdonald, F (1 November 2008). "Practice of prenatal diagnosis in the UK". Clinical Risk 14 (6): 218–221. doi:10.1258/cr.2008.080062.

Macfarquhar, Neil (December 19, 2008). "In a First, Gay Rights Are Pressed at the U.N". The New York Times.

Macklin R. Future challenges for the Declaration of Helsinki: Maintaining credibility in the face of ethical controversies. Address to Scientific Session, World Medical Association General Assembly, September 2003, Helsinki.

MacRae, Fiona (November 20, 2008). "Scientists are a step closer to creating 'elixir of life'". Daily Mail (London).

Maharishi Mahesh Yogi on the Bhagavad-Gita, a New Translation and Commentary, Chapter 1–6. Penguin Books, 1969, pp 94–95 (v 15)

Malik, Saurabh. "Torture main reason of death in police custody". The Tribune. Archived from the original on 31 March 2009. Retrieved 15 May 2011.

Managing Privacy: Information Technology and Corporate America - H. Jeff.

Mareike Meyn (December 9, 2008). "Beyond rights: Trading to win". COPLA. Archived from the original on April 29, 2011.

Marilyn M. Singleton (2014), The 'Science' of Eugenics: America's Moral Detour, Volume 19 Number 4 Winter 2014 (PDF), Journal of American Physicians and Surgeons, retrieved January 23, 2015.

Marshall Fredericks (2003). "GCVM History and Mission". Greater Cleveland Veteran's Memorial, Inc. Retrieved 2009-01-14.

Mary Rowe, "Options and choice for conflict resolution in the workplace" in Negotiation: Strategies for Mutual Gain, by Lavinia Hall (ed.), SAGE Publications, Inc., 1993, pp. 105–119.

Maspero, Henri. Translated by Frank A. Kierman, Jr. Taoism and Chinese Religion (University of Massachusetts Press, 1981), p. 211.

Masters, K. (2010), "Non-disclosure in Internet-based research: the risks explored through a case study", The Internet Journal of Medical Informatics 5 (2).

Mautner, Michael N. (2009). "Life-centered ethics, and the human future in space"(PDF). Bioethics 23: 433–440. doi:10.1111/j.1467-8519.2008.00688.x.PMID 19077128.

Mayer, Robert G. (2000-01-27). Embalming: History, Theory and Practice, 3rd ed., McGraw-Hill/Appleton and Lange. ISBN 978-0-8385-2187-8.

McManus, J., J; S. G. Mehta et al. (2005). "Informed consent and ethical issues in military medical research". Academic Emergency Medicine 12 (11): 1120–1126.doi:10.1111/j.1553-2712.2005.tb00839.x. PMID 16264083.

McWhorter, 2009: p. 204.

McWhorter, 2009: p. 205.

McWhorter, 2009: p. 377.

Medical.Webends.com > Double effect

Medical.Webends.com > Double effect Retrieved September 2010

Merchant, Brian. "125 Cities Passed Laws Placing Rights of Citizens, Nature Ahead of Corporations". Retrieved 29 October 2012.

Michel Weber and Will Desmond (eds.), Handbook of Whiteheadian Process Thought (Frankfurt/Lancaster, Ontos Verlag, Process Thought X1 and X2, 2008) and Ronny Desmet and Michel Weber (edited by), Whitehead., The Algebra of Metaphysics. Applied Process Metaphysics Summer Institute Memorandum, Louvain-la-Neuve, Les Éditions Chromatika, 2010.

More recently, the confidentiality laws have been changed so that doctors and nurses are under strict penalties if confidentiality is broken.

Motilal Tayade, Sunil Bhamare, Prathmesh Kambale, Kirankumar Jadhav, Doping in sports: Current review, International J of Current research and review, April 2013 ; 5(7) 83–86.

Moyn, Samuel (2010). The last utopia: human rights in history. Cambridge, Mass.: Belknap Press of Harvard University Press. ISBN 978-0-674-06434-8.

"Mrs R' and the human rights scripture". Asia Times (Hong Kong). November 2, 2002. Retrieved August 29, 2010.

Mughal, Muhammad Aurang Zeb. 2012. Spain. Steven L. Denver (ed.), Native Peoples of the World: An Encyclopedia of Groups, Cultures, and Contemporary Issues, Vol. 3. Armonk, NY: M.E. Sharpe, pp. 674–675.

Muzur, Amir (2014). "The nature of bioethics revisited: A comment on Tomislav Bracanoviæ". Developing World Bioethics 1: 109–110. doi:10.1111/dewb.12008.PMID 23279218.

"Myth busting". My family can overrule my decision to be a donor. Archived from the original on 22 May 2013.

Nader, Petkas, and Blackwell, Whistleblowing (1972).

Nancy Dickey, Kati Myllymäki, Judith Kazimirsky

Nancy S. Jecker, Medical futality, https://depts.washington. edu/bioethx/topics/futil.html Downloaded on 03/09/2015

National Academy of Sciences. 2009. On Being a Scientist: Third Edition. Washington, DC: The national Academies Press. Available at: http://www.nap.edu/catalog.php?record_ id=12192.

National Campaign for People's Right to Information (NCPRI)

National Conference of State Legislatures > Abortion Laws > Parental Involvement in Minors' Abortions

National Library of Medicine, 2006

National Museum American History. February 11, 2011. Retrieved July 14, 2011.

Nature's Economy (1994): A History of Ecological Ideas (Studies in Environment and History). Cambridge University Press. ISBN 0-521-46834-5.

Near, Janet P (Feb 1, 1985). "Organizational dissidence: The case of whistle-blowing".Journal of Business Ethics.

Nicholson, RH (2000). "If it ain't broke, don't fix it". Hastings Center Report 30 (1): 6.doi:10.2307/3527987. JSTOR 3527987. PMID 11645209.

Nicholson, RH; Crawley, FP (1999). "Revising the Declaration of Helsinki: a fresh start".Bulletin of medical ethics 151: 13–7. PMID 11657985.

Noyes, Nicole; Knopman, Jaime M.; Long, Kara; Coletta, Jaclyn M.; Abu-Rustum, Nadeem R. (2011). "Fertility considerations in the management of gynecologic malignancies". Gynecologic Oncology 120 (3): 326–33. doi:10.1016/j.ygyno.2010.09.012. PMID 20943258.

"OAS – Organization of American States: Democracy for peace, security, and development". Oas.org. Retrieved August 29, 2010.

On the legal history of eugenic sterilization in the U.S., see Paul Lombardo, "Eugenic Sterilization Laws", essay in the Eugenics Archive, available online athttp://www.eugenicsarchive. org/html/eugenics/essay8text.html.

Organ Donation Taskforce (2008). "The potential impact of an opt out system for organ donation in the UK" (PDF). United Kingdom: Department of Health. p. 22. Retrieved 8 March 2014.

"Osteopathic Oath". osteopathic.org. American Osteopathic Association. Retrieved 28 November 2014.

Page 100 of 'How to Make Good Decisions and Be Right All the Time', Iain King, Continuum, 2008, ISBN 978-1847-063-472.

Page 424 in:Tefferi, Ayalew (2001). Primary hematology. Totowa, NJ: Humana Press.ISBN 0-89603-664-2. [3]

Painter, Richard (2009), Getting the Government America Deserves: How Ethics Reform Can Make a Difference, Oxford University Press 978-0-19-537871-9

Palmer, Finlay, Martin, Victoria. "Faiths and Conservation: Buddhist Statement". Alliance of Religions and Conservation. Retrieved 3 December 2012.

Palmer, Finlay, Martin, Victoria. "Faiths and Ecology: What Does Jainism teach us about ecology?". Alliance of Religions and Conservation (ARC).

"Parents of UK's youngest organ donor hope others will be inspired". Retrieved April 24, 2015.

"Parliament panel backs Bill to keep parties out of RTI" Press Trust of India.

Peltier, James W., Anthony M. Allessandro, and Andrew J. Dahl. "Use of Social Media and College Student Organizations to Increase Support for Organ Donation and Advocacy: A Case Report." Progress in Transplantation (2012): 436–41. EBSCO. Web. 29 June 2014. Siminoff, Laura A., Amma A. Agyemang, and Heather M. Traino. "Consent to Organ Donation: A Review." Progress in Transplantation (2013): 99–104. EBSCO. Web.

Percival, Thomas (1849). Medical ethics. John Henry Parker. pp. 49–57 esp section 8 pg.52.

Peters (January 2001). "Torts II syllabus". University of Missouri-Columbia school of Law.

Philippe Letellier, chapter: History and Definition of a Word, in Euthanasia: Ethical and Human Aspects By Council of Europe.

Philippine Autonomy Act (Jones Law).

Pilgrim, David (2009-12-01). Key Concepts in Mental Health. p. 141.ISBN 9781848608801.

"Policies and Procedures of the Internal Audit Activity". City College of San Francisco. Retrieved July 7, 2011.

Policies regarding IRB members' industry relationships often lacking.

Pollard, B. J. (1993). "Autonomy and paternalism in medicine". The Medical Journal of Australia 159 (11–12): 797–802. PMID 8264472. edit

Posner, Richard A. (1983). The economics of justice (5. print ed.). Cambridge, Mass.: Harvard University Press. p. 271. ISBN 978-0674235267.

Press release, Office of the High Commissioner for Human Rights, United Nations, 27 August 2008.

Prince Albert v Strange (1848) 1 Mac. and G. 25

"Proclamation of Teheran". International Conference on Human Rights. 1968. Archived from the original on October 17, 2007. Retrieved November 8, 2007.

"Public Health". JAMA: the Journal of the American Medical Association (American Medical Association): 1138. June 6, 1896. doi:10.1001/jama.1896.02430750040011.

Punjab in Crisis: Human Rights in India (PDF). Human Rights Watch. 1990.

"Quebec end-of-life-care law means new era for health providers". Cbc.ca. Retrieved 8 June 2014.

Randall F. Ethical issues in cancer pain management. In: Sykes N, Bennett MI and Yuan C-S. Clinical pain management: Cancer pain. 2nd ed. London: Hodder Arnold; 2008. ISBN 978-0-340-94007-5. p. 93–100.

"Reconnecting the Dots — Reinterpreting Industry–Physician Relations — NEJM".

"Report 08: At a Glance". Amnesty International. 2008. Archived from the original on July 8, 2008. Retrieved October 22, 2008.

"Reproductive Rights are Human Rights" (PDF). UNFPA.

"Resveratrol may increase life span". Phytochemicals.info. Retrieved 2010-11-04.

"Revisiting the Commercial–Academic Interface — NEJM".

Riis P (July 1977). "Letter from...Denmark. Planning of scientific-ethical committees". British Medical Journal 2 (6080): 173–4. doi:10.1136/bmj.2.6080.173. PMC 1631019.PMID 871832.

Riis P. Perspectives on the fifth revision of the Declaration of Helsinki. JAMA 2000 Dec 20 284(23): 3045–6.

Rinèiæ, I., Muzur, A.: Fritz Jahr i raðanje europske bioetike (Fritz Jahr and the Birth of European Bioethics). Zagreb: Pergamena, 2012., page 141 (Croatian)

Robert A. Freitas Jr., Microbivores: Artificial Mechanical Phagocytes using Digest and Discharge Protocol, self-published, 2001 [4]

Robin Attfield, ed. (2003). Environmental ethics: an overview for the twenty-first century. Wiley-Blackwell. p. 17. ISBN 978-0-7456-2738-0.

Robinet, Isabelle. Taoism: Growth of a Religion (Stanford: Stanford University Press, 1997 [original French 1992]), p. 3–4.

Rosenbaum, Thane (2004). The Myth of Moral Justice. HarperCollins. pp. 247–248. ISBN 978-0-06-018816-0. Retrieved 2008-03-15.

Ross JS, Lackner JE, Lurie P, Gross CP, Wolfe S, Krumholz HM (2007). "Pharmaceutical company payments to physicians: early experiences with disclosure laws in Vermont and Minnesota". JAMA 297 (11): 1216–23. doi:10.1001/jama.297.11.1216.PMID 17374816.

R v Department of Health; Ex parte Source Informatics Ltd [2000] 1 All ER 786

Ryan CJ (2010). "Ethical issues, part 2: ethics, psychiatry, and end-of-life issues".Psychiatr Times 27 (6): 26–27.

Salganik, Matt. "After the Facebook emotional contagion experiment: A proposal for a positive path forward". Freedom to Tinker. Retrieved April 26, 2015.

Saltman Engineering Co. Ltd. v Campbell Engineering Co. Ltd. (1948) 65 R.P.C. 203

Samuel Moyn (author of book being reviewed), October 20, 2010, The New Republic, The Old New Thing, Retrieved Aug. 14, 2014

Sanderson, I. C.; Obeid, J. S.; Madathil, K. C.; Gerken, K.; Fryar, K.; Rugg, D.; Alstad, C. E.; Alexander, R.; Brady, K. T.; Gramopadhye, A. K.; Moskowitz, J. (2013). "Managing clinical research permissions electronically: A novel approach to enhancing recruitment and managing consents". Clinical Trials 10 (4): 604–611. doi:10.1177/1740774513491338.PMID 23785065.

Sanger, Margaret (1920). Woman and the New Race. Brentano. p. 100.

Sanger, Margaret (1922). The Pivot of Civilization. Brentano's. pp. 100–101. Nor do we believe that the community could or should send to the lethal chamber the defective progeny resulting from irresponsible and unintelligent breeding.

Schiffman and Robbins (2011). Green Issues and Debates: An A-to-Z Guide. SAGE Publications Inc. p. 32. ISBN 9781412996945.

"Scientists' Open Letter on Aging". Retrieved 20 April 2015.

Scott F. Gilbert (March 5, 2003). "Cheating Death: The Immortal Life Cycle ofTurritopsis". Developmental Biology, 8th edition. Retrieved 2007-04-02.

Security Council passes landmark resolution—world has responsibility to protect people from genocide Oxfam Press Release, April 28, 2006

"Security Recommendations For Stalking Victims". Privacyrights.org. Retrieved2012-01-01.

Selden, 2005: p. 206.

"Sexual orientation and gender identity". France Onu. Retrieved December 13, 2012.

Severson, Kim (9 December 2011). "Thousands Sterilized, a State Weighs Restitution". New York Times. Retrieved 10 December 2011.

Shafaat, Ahmad. "Ecology and the Teachings of the Prophets Muhammad and Jesus". Islamic Perspectives. Retrieved 1 December 2012.

Shafer-Landau, Russ. "The fundamentals of ethics." (2010). Pp 161

Shafer-Landau, Russ. "The fundamentals of ethics." (2010). Pp 163

Shaw 2008, p. 303.

Shaw SE, Petchey RP, Chapman J, Abbott S (2009). "A double-edged sword? Health research and research governance in UK primary care." Social Science and Medicine, 68: 912–918

"Should trade be considered a human right?". COPLA. December 9, 2008. Archived from the original on April 29, 2011.

Silva, Carlos (2011). "Biocentrism" in "Green Ethics and Philosophy: An A-to-Z Guide". Thousand Oaks, CA: SAGE Publications Inc. p. 55. ISBN 9781412996877.

Silva, Carlos (2011). "Biocentrism" in "Green Ethics and Philosophy: An A-to-Z Guide". Thousand Oaks, CA: SAGE Publications Inc. p. 56. ISBN 9781412996877.

Silva, Carlos (2011). "Biocentrism" in "Green Ethics and Philosophy: An A-to-Z Guide". Thousand Oaks, CA: SAGE Publications Inc. p. 57. ISBN 9781412996877.

Skovdal, M. and Abebe, T. (2012) "Reflexivity and dialogue: Addressing methodological and socio-ethical dilemmas in research with HIV-affected children in East Africa" Ethics, Policy and Environment 15(1):77–96

Smillie, Mark. "Biocentric (Life-Centered) Ethics". Carroll.edu. Retrieved 2 November 2012.

Sne•ana, Bošnjak (2001). "The declaration of Helsinki: The cornerstone of research ethics". Archive of Oncology 9 (3): 179–84.

Sokol, Daniel K. (2013). "'First do no harm' revisited". BMJ 347 (f6426). Retrieved 20 September 2014.

Solove 2008, p. 21.

Solove, Daniel J., Rotenberg, Marc, Schwartz, Paul M. Privacy, Information, and Technology, Aspen Publ. (2006) pp. 9–11

Stefansdottir, V; Skirton, H; Jonasson, K; Hardardottir, H; Jonsson, JJ (Jul 2010). "Effects of knowledge, education, and experience on acceptance of first trimester screening for chromosomal anomalies". Acta obstetricia et gynecologica Scandinavica 89(7): 931–8. doi:10.3109/00016341003686073. PMID 20235896.

Stern, 2005: pp. 27–31.

Stern, 2005: pp. 82–91.

Stern, 2005: pp. 84, 144.

Stern, Philip M. (1992). Still the Best Congress Money Can Buy. Regnery Gatgeway. pp. 168–176.

Stockhausen, K (2000). "The Declaration of Helsinki: revising ethical research guidelines for the 21st century". The Medical Journal of Australia 172 (6): 252–3. PMID 10860086.

"Stop Post-Firing Harassment Suits By Tracking And Investigating Every Complaint". HR Specialist: Minnesota Employment Law 2.11. 2009.

Subrahmaniam, Vidya (12 August 2013). "First-ever amendment to historic RTI Act tabled in Lok Sabha". The Hindu. Retrieved 1 December 2014.

Susan Currell (2006). Popular eugenics: national efficiency and American mass culture in the 1930s. Ohio University Press. pp. 2–3. ISBN 9780821416914. Retrieved July 18, 2011.

Swedlow A, Johnson G, Smithline N, Milstein A (1992). "Increased costs and rates of use in the California workers' compensation system as a result of self-referral by physicians". N Engl J Med 327 (21): 1502–6. doi:10.1056/NEJM199211193272-107. PMID 1406882.

Tabarrok, Alex (January 8, 2010). The Meat Market. The Wall Street Journal.

Table of Ratifications and Accessions.

Tassano, Fabian. The Power of Life or Death: Medical Coercion and the Euthanasia Debate. Foreword by Thomas Szasz, MD. London: Duckworth, 1995. Oxford: Oxford Forum, 1999.

Tayade MC, Karandikar PM, Role of Data Mining Techniques in Healthcare sector in India, Sch. J. App. Med. Sci., 2013; 1(3): June; 158–160.

Tayade MC, Kulkarni NB, The Interface of Technology and Medical Education in India: Current Trends and Scope. Indian Journal of Basic and Applied Medical Research; December 2011: Issue-1, Vol. 1, P. 8–12.

Tayade MC, Wankhede SV, Bhamare SB, Sabale BB, Role of image processing technology in healthcare sector: Review, International

Journal of Healthcare and Biomedical Research, 2(3), April 2014, Pages 8–11.

Tayade Motilal C, Latti Ramchandra G, Bioethics education in Preclinical medical curriculum: Review, International J. of Healthcare and Biomedical Research, Volume: 03, Issue: 04, July 2015, Pages 8–12.

Taylor, Paul (1986). Respect for Nature: A Theory of Environmental Ethics. Princeton University Press. p. 99. ISBN 978-0-691-02250-5.

Telstra Corp Ltd v First Netcom Pty Ltd (1997) 148 ALR 202 at 208.

Temkin, Owsei (2001). "On Second Thought". "On Second Thought" and Other Essays in the History of Medicine and Science. Johns Hopkins University. ISBN 978-0-8018-6774-3.

Temple R. Impact of the Declaration of Helsinki on medical research from a regulatory perspective. Address to the Scientific Session, World Medical Association General Assembly, September 2003.

Thaler, Richard H. (September 26, 2009). "Opting in vs. Opting Out". The New York Times. Archived from the original on March 8, 2014.

"The Bioethics Society of Ohio State". The bioethics society.org. ohio-state.edu. Retrieved 2013-09-17.

"The Great Purge". Cusd.chico.k12.ca.us. Retrieved August 29, 2010.

"The Hippocratic Oath Modern Version". University of California, San Diego.

The Indiana Supreme Court overturned the law in 1921 in Williams v. Smith, 131 NE 2 (Ind.), 1921, text at [3]

The International Human Rights Movement: Part of the Problem? Harvard Human Rights Journal / Vol. 15, Spring 2002.

"The law against slavery". Religion and ethics—ethical issues. BBC. Retrieved October 5, 2008.

"The Panama Pacific Exposition". Retrieved July 14, 2011.

The Psychiatry of Palliative Medicine: The Dying Mind, Page 209, Sandy Macleod.

The quotation is from Alan Westin.Westin, Alan F.; Blom-Cooper, Louis (1970). Privacy and freedom. London: Bodley Head. p. 7. ISBN 978-0370013251.

"The Role of the Yogyakarta Principles". International Gay and Lesbian Human Rights Commission. April 8, 2008.

"The Sanger-Hitler Equation", Margaret Sanger Papers Project Newsletter, #32, Winter 2002/3. New York University Department of History.

"Thursday's Fictions—Richard James Allen - Poems by book - Australian Poetry Library". Retrieved 20 April 2015.

Timmerman, Kelsey (2012). Where am I wearing?. California: Wiley.

Too Much Information: Informed Consent in Cultural Context. By Joseph J. Fins and Pablo Rodriguez del Pozo. Medscape 07/18/2011

Translated by Legge, James. The Texts of Taoism. 1962, Dover Press. NY.

"Transnational corporations should be held to human rights standards – UN expert". UN News Centre. October 13, 2003.

Tukufu Zuberi (2001). Thicker than blood: how racial statistics lie. University of Minnesota Press. p. 69. ISBN 9780816639090. Retrieved July 15, 2011.

Turkle S (1994). "Constructions and Reconstructions of Self in Virtual Reality". Mind, Culture, and Activity 1 (3): 158–167. doi:10.1080/10749039409524667.

Turkle S (1997). "Multiple subjectivity and virtual community at the end of the Freudian century". Sociological Inquiry 67 (1): 72–84. doi:10.1111/j.1475-682X.1997.tb00430.x.

Turnbull, George (1742). Observations Upon Liberal Education, In All Its Branches: In Three Parts. Millar.

Tyebkhan, G (2003). "Declaration of Helsinki: the ethical cornerstone of human clinical research". Indian journal of dermatology, venereology and leprology 69 (3): 245–7.PMID 17642902.

"United Nations Rights Council Page". United Nations News Page.

UNESCO. Universal Declaration on Bioethics and Human Rights. Adopted by the UNESCO General Conference at Paris, 19 October 2005.

"Vaccine Information Statement: Facts About VISs - Vaccines - CDC".http://www.cdc.gov. Centers for Disease Control and Prevention. Retrieved 30 July 2014.

"vallalar.org". vallalar.org. 2010-07-07. Retrieved 2010-11-04

Van Biema, David (February 7, 2008). "Christians Wrong About Heaven, Says Bishop ". Time. Retrieved May 5, 2010.

Vandekerckhove, Wim (2006). Whistleblowing and Organi-zational Social Responsibility: A Global Assessment. Ashgate.

Vanderpool, Harold Y. (1996). The Ethics of Research Involving Human Subjects: Facing the 21st Century. Frederick, Maryland: University Publishing Group, Inc. p. 85. ISBN 1-55572-036-6

Vanderpool, Harold Y. (1996). The Ethics of Research Involving Human Subjects: Facing the 21st Century. Frederick, Maryland: University Publishing Group, Inc. pp. 433–436.ISBN 1-55572-036-6.

Voluntary and involuntary euthanasia BBC Accessed 12 February 2012. Archived from the original here.

Vuletic, Mark. "Philosophy Notes: Singer, "All Animals Are Equal"". vuletic.com. Retrieved 8 November 2012.

Walker, Peter (1991). International Search and Rescue Teams, A League Discussion Paper. Geneva: League of the Red Cross and Red Crescent Societies.

Walter, Klein eds, The Story of Bioethics: From seminal works to contemporary explorations.

Ward, Martha C. (1986). Poor Women, Powerful Men: America's Great Experiment in Family Planning. Boulder: Westview Press. p. 95.

Watson, James D.; Berry, Andrew (2003). DNA: The Secret of Life. Alfred A. Knopf. pp. 29–31. ISBN 0-375-41546-7.

Watts, Duncan. "Stop complaining about the Facebook study. It's a golden age for research". The Guardian. Retrieved April 26, 2015.

Wazana A (2000). "Physicians and the pharmaceutical industry: is a gift ever just a gift?".JAMA 283 (3): 373–80. doi:10.1001/jama.283.3.373. PMID 10647801.

"Whistleblowing". Retrieved 2015-05-06.

"WHO | Informed Consent Form Templates". who.int. Retrieved 14 September 2014.

"Why Privacy is Important". Philosophy and Public Affairs 4 (4): 323–333 (Summer 1975).

Williams v. Smith, 131 NE 2 (Ind.), 1921, text at

Williams, G.C. 1957. Pleiotropy, natural selection and the evolution of senescence.Evolution, 11:398-411. [2] Paper in which Williams describes his theory of antagonistic pleiotropy.

Wilson, Ralph F. "Peacock as an Ancient Christian Symbol of Eternal Life". Jesus Walk Bible Study Series. Retrieved January 18, 2011.

WMA Medical Ethics Committee. Updating the WMA Declaration of Helsinki. Wld Med J 1999 45: 11–13.

"World Day against Death Penalty". ILGA. Retrieved August 29, 2010.

WMA Press Release: WMA revises the Declaration of Helsinki. 9 October 2000

World Medical Association, Inc. "WMA History". www.wma.net. World Medical Association, Inc. Retrieved 1 November 2014.

World Medical Association. Proposed revision of the Declaration of Helsinki Document 17.C/Rev1/99

World Medical, Association (1999). "Proposed revision of the Declaration of Helsinki". Bulletin of medical ethics 147: 18–22. PMID 11657218.

World Report 2014 (PDF). Human Rights Watch. 2014. pp. 334–341.

Worsnip, Patrick (December 18, 2008). "U.N. divided over gay rights declaration". Reuters. Retrieved August 29, 2010.

Worster, Donald (1994). Nature's Economy: A History of Ecological Ideas (Studies in Environment and History). Cambridge University Press. ISBN 0-521-46834-5.

www.wikipedia.com

"Yahoo Education". Education.yahoo.com. Retrieved 2012-07-08.

Yu, Lei, Mouchang, Yi (2009). "13. Biocentric Ethical Theories". Environment and Development - Vol. II (PDF). China. p. 422. ISBN 978-1-84826-721-3.

Zavales, Anastasios (December 10, 1993). "Genital mutilation and the United Nations". National Organization of Circumcision Information Resource Centers. Retrieved August 29, 2010.

Zemskaya, E. A. (9 April 2005). "Ocj, tyyjcnb heccrjq htxb"vbuhfynjd xtndthnjq djkys (Features of the Russian language of fourth wave immigrants)" (in Russian). Gramota.ru. Retrieved 24 February 2009.

Ziegler, Mary (2008). "Eugenic Feminism: Mental Hygiene, The Women's Movement, And The Campaign For Eugenic Legal Reform, 1900–1935". Harvard Journal of Law and Gender31 (1): 211–236.

Index